Pharmacology

Editor

ALAN D. KAYE

ANESTHESIOLOGY CLINICS

www.anesthesiology.theclinics.com

Consulting Editor
LEE A. FLEISHER

June 2017 • Volume 35 • Number 2

ELSEVIER

1600 John F. Kennedy Boulevard • Suite 1800 • Philadelphia, Pennsylvania, 19103-2899

http://www.theclinics.com

ANESTHESIOLOGY CLINICS Volume 35, Number 2
June 2017 ISSN 1932-2275, ISBN-13: 978-0-323-52997-6

Editor: Katie Pfaff
Developmental Editor: Kristen Helm

Anesthesiology Clinics (ISSN 1932-2275) is published quarterly by Elsevier Inc., 360 Park Avenue South, New York, NY 10010-1710. Months of issue are March, June, September, and December. Periodicals postage paid at New York, NY and at additional mailing offices. Subscription prices are $100.00 per year (US student/resident), $333.00 per year (US individuals), $404.00 per year (Canadian individuals), $620.00 per year (US institutions), $783.00 per year (Canadian institutions), $225.00 per year (Canadian and foreign student/resident), $460.00 per year (foreign individuals), and $783.00 per year (foreign institutions). To receive student and resident rate, orders must be accompanied by name of affiliated institution, date of term, and the *signature* of program/residency coordinator on institutions letterhead. Orders will be billed at individual rate until proof of status is received. Foreign air speed delivery is included in all *Clinics'* subscription prices. All prices are subject to change without notice. POSTMASTER: Send address changes to *Anesthesiology Clinics,* Elsevier Health Sciences Division, Subscription Customer Service, 3251 Riverport Lane, Maryland Heights, MO 63043. Customer Service (orders, claims, online, change of address): Elsevier Health Sciences Division, Subscription Customer Service, 3251 Riverport Lane, Maryland Heights, MO 63043. **Tel:1-800-654-2452 (U.S. and Canada); 314-447-8871 (outside U.S. and Canada). Fax: 314-447-8029. E-mail: journalscustomerservice-usa@elsevier.com (for print support); journalsonlinesupport-usa@elsevier.com (for online support).**

Reprints. For copies of 100 or more of articles in this publication, please contact the Commercial Reprints Department, Elsevier Inc., 360 Park Avenue South, New York, NY 10010-1710. Tel.: 212-633-3874; Fax: 212-633-3820; E-mail: reprints@elsevier.com.

Anesthesiology Clinics, is also published in Spanish by McGraw-Hill Inter-americana Editores S. A., P.O. Box 5-237, 06500 Mexico D. F., Mexico.

Anesthesiology Clinics, is covered in *MEDLINE/PubMed (Index Medicus), Current Contents/Clinical Medicine, Excerpta Medica, ISI/BIOMED*, and *Chemical Abstracts*.

Contributors

CONSULTING EDITOR

LEE A. FLEISHER, MD, FACC
Robert D. Dripps Professor and Chair of Anesthesiology and Critical Care, Professor of Medicine, Perelman School of Medicine, University of Pennsylvania, Philadelphia, Pennsylvania

EDITOR

ALAN D. KAYE, MD, PhD, DABA, DABPM, DABIPP
Professor, Program Director and Chairman, Department of Anesthesiology, Director, Pain Services, Hospital Director of Anesthesia, University Medical Center Hospital, Professor, Department of Pharmacology, Louisiana State University School of Medicine T6M5, Professor of Anesthesia and Pharmacology, Tulane School of Medicine, New Orleans, Louisiana

AUTHORS

CAMELLIA ASGARIAN, MD
Department of Anesthesiology, Louisiana State University School of Medicine, New Orleans, Louisiana

DANIEL BANG, MD
Department of Anesthesiology, Harbor-UCLA Medical Center, Torrance, California

BURTON D. BEAKLEY, MD
Department of Anesthesiology, Tulane School of Medicine, New Orleans, Louisiana

SASCHA S. BEUTLER, MD, PhD
Department of Anesthesiology, Perioperative and Pain Medicine, Brigham and Women's Hospital, Harvard Medical School, Boston, Massachusetts

ANAIR BEVERLY, MBBS, BSc, MRCP
Department of Anesthesiology, Perioperative and Pain Medicine, Brigham and Women's Hospital, Boston, Massachusetts

KARISHMA PATEL BHANGARE, MD
Department of Anesthesiology, Perioperative and Pain Medicine, Brigham and Women's Hospital, Harvard Medical School, Boston, Massachusetts

LARA K. BONASERA, MD
Staff Anesthesiologist, Department of Anesthesiology, Advocate Illinois Masonic Medical Center, Chicago, Illinois

GREGORY J. BORDELON, MD
Assistant Professor, Department of Anesthesiology, Louisiana State University Medical Center, New Orleans, Louisiana

REZA M. BORNA, MD
Assistant Professor of Anesthesiology, Department of Anesthesiology and Perioperative Medicine, David Geffen School of Medicine at UCLA, Ronald Reagan UCLA Medical Center, Los Angeles, California

ANDREW BRUNK, MD
Department of Anesthesiology, Louisiana State University School of Medicine, New Orleans, Louisiana

KENNETH D. CANDIDO, MD
Chairman and Professor, Department of Anesthesiology and Pain Medicine, Advocate Illinois Masonic Medical Center, Departments of Anesthesiology and Surgery, University of Illinois, Chicago, Illinois

CATHERINE M. CHA, MD
Assistant Clinical Professor, Department of Anesthesiology and Perioperative Medicine, David Geffen School of Medicine at UCLA, Los Angeles, California

JOHN CHALABI, MD
Department of Anesthesiology and Perioperative Medicine, David Geffen School of Medicine at UCLA, Los Angeles, California

DEBBIE CHANDLER, MD
Department of Anesthesiology, Louisiana State University Health, Shreveport, Louisiana

DANIEL CHANG, MD
Department of Anesthesiology, Yale University School of Medicine, New Haven, Connecticut

LYNN O. CHOI, MD
Assistant Clinical Professor, Department of Anesthesiology and Perioperative Medicine, David Geffen School of Medicine at UCLA, Los Angeles, California

RICHARD C. CLARKE, MD
Department of Anesthesiology, Louisiana State University Health Sciences Center, New Orleans, Louisiana

ELYSE M. CORNETT, PhD
Assistant Professor of Research and Clinical Research Coordinator, Department of Anesthesiology, Louisiana State University Health Science Center, Louisiana State University School of Medicine, New Orleans, Louisiana; Department of Anesthesiology, Louisiana State University Health, Shreveport, Louisiana

JUSTIN B. CREEL, MD
Department of Anesthesiology, Louisiana State University School of Medicine, Shreveport, Louisiana

NICHOLAS DARENSBURG, MD
Department of Anesthesiology, Louisiana State University School of Medicine, Shreveport, Louisiana

JAMES H. DIAZ, MD, DrPH
Department of Anesthesiology and School of Public Health, Louisiana State University Health Science Center, New Orleans, Louisiana

KEN P EHRHARDT Jr, MD
Department of Anesthesiology, Louisiana State University Health Science Center, New Orleans, Louisiana

AMIR O. ELHASSAN, MD
Department of Anesthesiology, Louisiana State University Health Sciences Center, New Orleans, Louisiana

CHARLES J. FOX, MD
Professor and Chairman, Department of Anesthesiology, Louisiana State University Health-Shreveport, Shreveport, Louisiana

JEREMY B. GREEN, MD
Resident, Department of Anesthesiology, Louisiana State University Health Science Center-New Orleans, New Orleans, Louisiana

KARINA GRITSENKO, MD
Program Director, Regional Anesthesia and Acute Pain Medicine Fellowship, Director, Regional Anesthesia and Acute Pain Medicine Resident Rotations, Assistant Professor of Anesthesiology, Family & Social Medicine, and Physical Medicine & Rehabilitation, Montefiore Medical Center, Bronx, New York

JOSEPH R. GUENZER, MD
Assistant Professor, Department of Anesthesiology, University of Utah Medical School, Salt Lake City, Utah

BRENDON HART, DO
Resident, Department of Anesthesiology, Louisiana State University School of Medicine-Shreveport, Shreveport, Louisiana

ERIK M. HELANDER, MBBS
Department of Anesthesiology, Louisiana State University School of Medicine, New Orleans, Louisiana

RICHARD W. HONG, MD
Associate Clinical Professor and Chief of Obstetric Anesthesiology; Department of Anesthesiology and Perioperative Medicine, David Geffen School of Medicine at UCLA, Los Angeles, California

DORA HSU, MD
Department of Anesthesiology, Harbor-UCLA Medical Center, Torrance, California

ERIC HSU, MD
Department of Anesthesiology and Perioperative Medicine, David Geffen School of Medicine at UCLA, Los Angeles, California

JONATHAN S. JAHR, MD
Professor Emeritus, Department of Anesthesiology and Perioperative Medicine, David Geffen School of Medicine at UCLA, Ronald Reagan UCLA Medical Center, Los Angeles, California

PREYA JHITA, MD
Department of Anesthesiology, Louisiana State University School of Medicine, New Orleans, Louisiana

INDERJEET JULKA, MD
Department of Anesthesiology, Harbor-UCLA Medical Center, Torrance, California

ALICE KAI, BA
Department of Anesthesiology, Yale University School of Medicine, New Haven, Connecticut

MUDIT KAUSHAL, MD
Resident, Department of Anesthesiology, Montefiore Medical Center, Bronx, New York

ALAN D. KAYE, MD, PhD, DABA, DABPM, DABIPP
Professor, Program Director and Chairman, Department of Anesthesiology, Director, Pain Services, Hospital Director of Anesthesia, University Medical Center Hospital, Professor, Department of Pharmacology, Louisiana State University School of Medicine T6M5, Professor of Anesthesia and Pharmacology, Tulane School of Medicine, New Orleans, Louisiana

CHIH H. KING, MD, PhD
Department of Anesthesiology, Perioperative and Pain Medicine, Brigham and Women's Hospital, Boston, Massachusetts

SUSANNA KMIECIK, MD
Department of Anesthesiology and Perioperative Medicine, CA 3 Resident, David Geffen School of Medicine at UCLA, Ronald Reagan UCLA Medical Center, Los Angeles, California

NEBOJSA NICK KNEZEVIC, MD, PhD
Vice Chair for Research and Education and Associate Professor, Department of Anesthesiology and Pain Medicine, Advocate Illinois Masonic Medical Center, Departments of Anesthesiology and Surgery, University of Illinois, Chicago, Illinois

ALLYSON LEMAY, MD
Department of Anesthesiology, Perioperative and Pain Medicine, Harvard Medical School, Brigham and Women's Hospital, Boston, Massachusetts

HENRY LIU, MD
Department of Anesthesiology & Perioperative Medicine, Hahnemann University Hospital, Drexel University College of Medicine, Philadelphia, Pennsylvania

OLLE LJUNGQVIST, MD, PhD
Professor of Surgery, Chairman ERAS Society, Faculty of Medicine and Health, Department of Surgery, School of Health and Medical Sciences, Örebro University, Örebro, Sweden

KEN F. MANCUSO, MD
Assistant Professor, Associate Program Director, Department of Anesthesiology, Louisiana State University Health Science Center, New Orleans, Louisiana

JOSEPH MELTZER, MD
Associate Professor, Department of Anesthesiology, David Geffen School of Medicine, University of California, Los Angeles, Los Angeles, California

BETHANY MENARD, MD
Department of Anesthesiology, Louisiana State University School of Medicine, New Orleans, Louisiana

NATALE Z. NAIM, MD
Department of Anesthesiology and Perioperative Medicine, David Geffen School of Medicine at UCLA, Los Angeles, California

VIET NGUYEN, MD
Assistant Clinical Professor, Department of Anesthesiology, Louisiana State University Health Science Center-New Orleans, New Orleans, Louisiana

MATTHEW B. NOVITCH, BS
Medical Student, Medical College of Wisconsin, Wausau, Wisconsin

IRA W. PADNOS, MD
Department of Anesthesiology, Louisiana State University Health Science Center, New Orleans, Louisiana

JACQUELYN R. PAETZOLD, DO
Department of Anesthesiology, Tulane School of Medicine, New Orleans, Louisiana

EDWARD PARK, MD
Assistant Clinical Professor of Anesthesiology, Department of Anesthesiology and Perioperative Medicine, Ronald Regan UCLA Medical Center, Los Angeles, California

SHILPADEVI PATIL, MD
Department of Anesthesiology, Louisiana State University Health-Shreveport, Shreveport, Louisiana

OSCAR J. PEROZO, MD
Clinical Research Fellow, Department of Anesthesiology, Advocate Illinois Masonic Medical Center, Chicago, Illinois

MAUNAK V. RANA, MD
Clinical Associate Professor, Department of Anesthesiology, Advocate Illinois Masonic Medical Center, Chicago, Illinois

XIULU RUAN, MD
Adjunct Clinical Associate Professor of Anesthesia, Department of Anesthesiology, Louisiana State University Health Science Center, New Orleans, Louisiana

RYAN E. RUBIN, MD, MPH
Assistant Professor, Department of Anesthesiology, Louisiana State University School of Medicine, New Orleans, Louisiana

RAMSEY SABA, MD
Department of Anesthesiology, Perioperative and Pain Medicine, Brigham and Women's Hospital, Harvard Medical School, Boston, Massachusetts

ALI SALEHI, MD
Associate Clinical Professor of Anesthesiology, Department of Anesthesiology and Perioperative Medicine, Ronald Regan UCLA Medical Center, Los Angeles, California

SUDIPTA SEN, MD
Department of Anesthesiology, Louisiana State University Health-Shreveport, Shreveport, Louisiana

SUMIT SINGH, MD
Department of Anesthesiology, David Geffen School of Medicine at UCLA, Los Angeles, California

MARIAH KINCAID TANIOUS, MD, MPH
Department of Anesthesiology, Perioperative and Pain Medicine, Brigham and Women's Hospital, Harvard Medical School, Boston, Massachusetts

DAWN TIEMANN, MD
Assistant Clinical Professor, Department of Anesthesiology, Louisiana State University Health Science Center-New Orleans, New Orleans, Louisiana

LIEN B. TRAN, MD
Department of Anesthesiology, Louisiana State University Health Sciences Center, New Orleans, Louisiana

THOMAS N. TRANG, MD
Department of Anesthesiology, Tulane School of Medicine, New Orleans, Louisiana

RICHARD D. URMAN, MD, MBA
Department of Anesthesiology, Perioperative and Pain Medicine, Brigham and Women's Hospital, Harvard Medical School, Boston, Massachusetts

NALINI VADIVELU, MD
Associate Professor, Department of Anesthesiology, Yale University School of Medicine, New Haven, Connecticut

CRISTIANNA VALLERA, MD
Assistant Clinical Professor, Department of Anesthesiology and Perioperative Medicine, David Geffen School of Medicine at UCLA, Los Angeles, California

SIMON WILLIS, MD
Resident Physician, Department of Physical Medicine and Rehabilitation, MedStar Georgetown University Hospital/National Rehabilitation Hospital, Washington, DC

Contents

Foreword: Pharmacology **xvii**

Lee A. Fleisher

Preface: The Future of Pharmacology in Anesthesia Practice **xix**

Alan D. Kaye

Ketorolac, Oxymorphone, Tapentadol, and Tramadol: A Comprehensive Review **e1**

Nalini Vadivelu, Daniel Chang, Erik M. Helander, Gregory J. Bordelon, Alice Kai, Alan D. Kaye, Dora Hsu, Daniel Bang, and Inderjeet Julka

Pain remains a tremendous burden on patients and for the health care system, with uncontrolled pain being the leading cause of disability in this country. There are a variety of medications that can be used in the treatment of pain, including ketorolac, oxymorphone, tapentadol, and tramadol. Depending on the clinical situation, these drugs can be used as monotherapy or in conjunction with other types of medications in a multimodal approach. A strong appreciation of pharmacologic properties of these agents and potential side effects is warranted for clinicians.

Anticoagulation and Neuraxial/Peripheral Anesthesia **e21**

Mudit Kaushal, Ryan E. Rubin, Alan D. Kaye, and Karina Gritsenko

Novel anticoagulants (NAGs) have emerged as the preferred alternatives to vitamin K antagonists. In patients being considered for regional anesthesia, these drugs present a layer of complexity in the preprocedure evaluation. There are no established tests to monitor anticoagulant activity and our experience is short with these drugs. These authors believe it is important to review the relevant hematology, orthopedics, and anesthesiology literature to provide a valuable reference for the clinician who is met with these challenges. In addition to discussing NAGs, we also review the existing American Society of Regional Anesthesia guidelines for heparin, low-molecular-weight heparin, and antiplatelet agents.

Pharmacology of Antiemetics: Update and Current Considerations in Anesthesia Practice **e41**

Alan D. Kaye, Elyse M. Cornett, John Chalabi, Natale Z. Naim, Matthew B. Novitch, Justin B. Creel, Preya Jhita, Thomas N. Trang, Jacquelyn R. Paetzold, Nicholas Darensburg, Burton D. Beakley, and Richard D. Urman

Postoperative nausea and vomiting (PONV) is associated with delayed recovery and dissatisfaction after surgical procedures. A key component to management is identifying risk factors and high-risk populations. Advances in pharmacologic therapeutics have resulted in agents targeting different pathways associated with the mediation of nausea and vomiting.

This review focuses on these agents and the clinical aspects of their use in patients postoperatively. Combination therapies are reviewed, and studies demonstrate that when 2 or more antiemetic agents acting on different receptors are used, an overall improved efficacy is demonstrated when compared with a single agent alone in patients.

Total Parenteral and Enteral Nutrition in the ICU: Evolving Concepts **181**

Amir O. Elhassan, Lien B. Tran, Richard C. Clarke, Sumit Singh, and Alan D. Kaye

Appropriate nutrition in the hospital setting, particularly in critically ill patients, has long been tied to improving clinical outcomes. During critical illness, inflammatory mediators and cytokines lead to the creation of a catabolic state to facilitate the use of endogenous energy sources to meet increased energy demands. This process results in increasing the likelihood of overfeeding. The literature has revealed exponential advances in understanding the molecular basis of nutritional support and evolution of clinical protocols aimed at treating artificial nutritional support as a therapeutic intervention, preventing loss of lean body mass and metabolic deterioration to improve clinical outcomes in the critically ill.

Anticoagulant Reversal and Anesthetic Considerations **191**

Joseph Meltzer and Joseph R. Guenzer

Bleeding complications are a common concern with the use of anticoagulant agents. In many situations, reversing of neutralizing their effects may be warranted. Prothrombin complex concentrate replaces coagulation factors lowered by warfarin, as does fresh frozen plasma, but in a more concentrated form. Protamine negates the effect of heparin and combines chemically with heparin molecules to form an inactive salt. It also partially reverses the effects of low-molecular-weight heparin. Recombinant activated factor VII is a nonspecific procoagulant that activates the extrinsic clotting pathway, resulting in thrombin generation, but does not directly neutralize the activity of any of the new oral anticoagulants.

An Update on Nonopioids: Intravenous or Oral Analgesics for Perioperative Pain Management **e55**

Alan D. Kaye, Elyse M. Cornett, Erik Helander, Bethany Menard, Eric Hsu, Brendon Hart, and Andrew Brunk

Despite an appreciation for many unwanted physiologic effects from inadequate postoperative pain relief, moderate to severe postoperative pain remains commonplace. Although treatment options have evolved in recent years, the use of nonopioid analgesics agents can reduce acute pain-associated morbidity and mortality. This review focuses on the importance of effective postoperative nonopioid analgesic agents, such as acetaminophen, nonsteroidal anti-inflammatory agents, gabapentinoid agents, NMDA antagonists, alpha 2 agonists, and steroids, in opioid sparing and enhancing recovery. A careful literature review focusing on these treatment options, potential benefits, and side effects associated with these strategies is emphasized in this review.

Uterotonic Medications: Oxytocin, Methylergonovine, Carboprost, Misoprostol 207

Cristianna Vallera, Lynn O. Choi, Catherine M. Cha, and Richard W. Hong

Uterine atony is a common cause of primary postpartum hemorrhage, which remains a major cause of pregnancy-related mortality for women worldwide. Oxytocin, methylergonovine, carboprost, and misoprostol are commonly used to restore uterine tone. Oxytocin is the first-line agent. Methylergonovine and carboprost are both highly effective second-line agents with severe potential side effects. Recent studies have called into question the effectiveness of misoprostol as an adjunct to other uterotonic agents, but it remains a useful therapeutic in resource-limited practice environments. We review the current role these medications play in the prevention and treatment of uterine atony.

Pulmonary Vasodilators and Anesthesia Considerations 221

Jeremy B. Green, Brendon Hart, Elyse M. Cornett, Alan D. Kaye, Ali Salehi, and Charles J. Fox

Pulmonary hypertension (PH) is a complex disease process of the pulmonary vasculature system characterized by elevated pulmonary arterial pressures. Patients with PH are at increased risk for morbidity and mortality, including intraoperatively and postoperatively. Appreciation by the clinical anesthesiologist of the pathophysiology of PH is warranted. Careful and meticulous strategy using appropriate anesthetic medications, pulmonary vasodilator and inotropic agents, and careful fluid management all increase the likelihood of the best possible outcome in this challenging patient population.

Alpha-2 Agonists 233

Viet Nguyen, Dawn Tiemann, Edward Park, and Ali Salehi

Alpha-2 adrenergic receptors are spread throughout the central and peripheral nervous system, specifically in the pontine locus coeruleus, medullospinal tracts, rostral ventrolateral medulla, and the dorsal horn of the spinal cord. Alpha-2 agonist agents cause neuromodulation in these centers, leading to sedation, analgesia, vasodilatation, and bradycardia with little effect on the respiratory drive, which accounts for their good safety profile. The 2 major drugs in this group are clonidine and dexmedetomidine. Their clinical applications in anesthesia practice include providing sedation in the intensive care unit or for minor procedures, adjuvant to general and regional anesthesia, analgesia, and as premedicating agents.

Perioperative Pharmacologic Considerations in Obesity 247

Simon Willis, Gregory J. Bordelon, and Maunak V. Rana

Obesity has increased in incidence worldwide. Along with the increased number of obese patients, comorbid conditions are also more prevalent in this population. Obesity leads to changes in the physiology of patients along with an altered response to pharmacologic therapy. Vigilant perioperative physicians must be aware of the unique characteristics of administered agents in order to appropriately provide anesthetic care for obese patients. Because of the variability in tissue content in obese patients and changes in pharmacokinetic modeling, a one-size-fits-all approach is not justified and a more sophisticated and prudent approach is indicated.

Pharmacologic Considerations of Anesthetic Agents in Geriatric Patients 259

Maunak V. Rana, Lara K. Bonasera, and Gregory J. Bordelon

Aging is a natural process of declining organ function and reserve. Census data show that the geriatric population is expected to grow to nearly 30%. More than half of geriatric patients have 1 or more surgical procedures in their lifetimes. Moreover, this is the population at greatest risk of morbidity and mortality with any given complication. There is remarkable variability in health across the age spectrum, from fit to frail and compromised. This variability requires a unique approach to anesthetic delivery and drug dosing on an individual basis to avoid complications such as postoperative cognitive dysfunction and delirium.

Pharmacologic Considerations of Anesthetic Agents in Pediatric Patients: A Comprehensive Review e73

Alan D. Kaye, Charles J. Fox, Ira W. Padnos, Ken P Ehrhardt Jr, James H. Diaz, Elyse M. Cornett, Debbie Chandler, Sudipta Sen, and Shilpadevi Patil

Acute pain in the pediatric population has important differences in terms of biology, intrapopulation variation, and epidemiology. Discussion as to the pharmacologic considerations of anesthetic agents, such as induction agents, neuromuscular blockers, opioids, local anesthetics, and adjuvant agents, is presented in this article. Special considerations and concerns, such as risk for propofol infusion syndrome and adverse potential side effects of anesthesia agents, are discussed. Anesthesiologists managing pediatric patients need to have a firm understanding of physiologic and pharmacologic differences compared with the adult population. Future studies to improve the understanding of pharmacokinetics in the pediatric population are needed.

Cardiovascular Pharmacology: An Update and Anesthesia Considerations 273

Camellia Asgarian, Henry Liu, and Alan D. Kaye

Cardiovascular disease remains a leading cause of morbidity and mortality worldwide. The development of therapeutic agents for the treatment of cardiovascular diseases has always been a priority because of the huge potential market for these drugs. These medications should be part of the anesthesiologist's armamentarium because the typical surgical patient is older and has more comorbidities than in the past. This article reviews commonly used cardiovascular medications that are important in managing patients with unstable hemodynamics.

Pharmacogenomics in Anesthesia 285

Ramsey Saba, Alan D. Kaye, and Richard D. Urman

A significant number of commonly administered medications in anesthesia show wide clinical interpatient variability. Some of these include neuromuscular blockers, opioids, local anesthetics, and inhalation anesthetics. Individual genetic makeup may account for and predict cardiovascular outcomes after cardiac surgery. These interactions can manifest at any

concerning, multisystemic, long-term, and short-term side effects, which increase morbidity and prolong admissions. Enhanced recovery is a systematic process addressing each aspect affecting recovery. This article outlines the evidence base forming the current multimodal analgesia recommendations made by the Enhanced Recovery After Surgery Society (ERAS). We describe current evidence and important future directions for effective perioperative multimodal analgesia in enhanced recovery pathways.

Pharmacologic Properties of Novel Local Anesthetic Agents in Anesthesia Practice **315**

Chih H. King, Sascha S. Beutler, Alan D. Kaye, and Richard D. Urman

Therapeutic duration of traditional local anesthetics when used in peripheral nerve blocks is normally limited. This article describes novel approaches to extend the duration of peripheral nerve blocks currently available or in development. Three newer approaches on extending the duration of peripheral nerve blocks include site-1 sodium channel blockers, novel local anesthetics delivery systems, and novel adjuvants of local anesthetics. Compared with plain amide-based and ester-based local anesthetics, alternative approaches show significant promise in decreasing postoperative pain, rescue opioid requirement, hospital length-of-stay, and overall health care cost, without compromising the established safety profile of traditional local anesthetics.

Pharmacology of Acetaminophen, Nonsteroidal Antiinflammatory Drugs, and Steroid Medications: Implications for Anesthesia or Unique Associated Risks **e145**

Kenneth D. Candido, Oscar J. Perozo, and Nebojsa Nick Knezevic

Acetaminophen, nonsteroidal antiinflammatory drugs (NSAIDs), and corticosteroids, historically used in perioperative management, are potent analgesic medications. They primarily inhibit the cyclooxygenase (COX) enzyme, decreasing the synthesis of prostaglandins, and modulating pain and temperature. Acetaminophen does not inhibit this synthesis at the inflammatory site. The primary mechanism of action of corticosteroids involves regulation of nuclear expression of genes involved in inflammatory pathways and other systemic effects. Metaanalyses have added purposeful perioperative indications, clarified misconceptions, and established protocols for administering these drugs. Some indications, doses, clinical considerations, and adverse effects need to be further studied.

Pharmacology of Octreotide: Clinical Implications for Anesthesiologists and Associated Risks **327**

Reza M. Borna, Jonathan S. Jahr, Susanna Kmiecik, Ken F. Mancuso, and Alan D. Kaye

Many patients presenting with a history of foregut, midgut neuroendocrine tumors (NETs) or carcinoid syndrome can experience life-threatening carcinoid crises during anesthesia or surgery. Clinicians should understand the pharmacology of octreotide and appreciate the use of continuous infusions of high-dose octreotide, which can minimize intraoperative carcinoid crises. We administer a prophylactic 500-μg bolus of octreotide intravenously (IV) and begin a continuous infusion of 500 μg/h for all NET patients. Advantages include low cost and excellent safety profile. High-dose octreotide for midgut and foregut NETs requires an appreciation of the pathophysiology involved in the disease, pharmacology, drug–drug interactions, and side effects.

Revisiting Oxycodone Analgesia: A Review and Hypothesis **e163**

Xiulu Ruan, Ken F. Mancuso, and Alan D. Kaye

Oxycodone, a semisynthetic opioid analgesic, is widely used in clinical practice. Oxycodone and morphine seem to be equally effective and equipotent; however, morphine is 10 times more potent than oxycodone when given epidurally. This article provides an updated review of the basic pharmacology of oxycodone with a special focus on pharmacokinetic/pharmacodynamics properties. The controversy regarding oxycodone-mediated effects for visceral pain via agonism and the possible role of peripheral opioid analgesia are discussed in the present investigation in an attempt to propose a plausible explanation to the perplexing question of oxycodone analgesia.

An Analysis of New Approaches and Drug Formulations for Treatment of Chronic Low Back Pain **341**

Karishma Patel Bhangare, Alan D. Kaye, Nebojsa Nick Knezevic, Kenneth D. Candido, and Richard D. Urman

The prevalence of chronic low back pain (CLBP) is increasing. Treatment is effective in less than 50% of patients after 1 year. This review investigates new treatments for CLBP. An extensive literature review focuses on new treatments for CLBP. Their safety and efficacy were evaluated and are described in detail in this review. The investigation identified new treatments for CLBP including chemonucleolysis, platelet-rich plasma injections, artemin, tanezumab, and stem cells. Further research and innovation are needed to implement these methods into practice and assess clinical significance. The current evidence suggests that there are promising new agents for the treatment of CLBP.

Index **351**

ANESTHESIOLOGY CLINICS

FORTHCOMING ISSUES

September 2017
Transplantation
Christopher Wray and Aman Mahajan, *Editors*

December 2017
Anesthesia Outside the Operating Room
Mark S. Weiss and Wendy L. Gross, *Editors*

March 2018
Quality Improvement and Implementation Science
Meghan Lane-Fall, *Editor*

RECENT ISSUES

March 2017
Obstetric Anesthesia
Onyi C. Onuoha and Robert R. Gaiser, *Editors*

December 2016
Medically Complex Patients
Robert B. Schonberger and Stanley H. Rosenbaum, *Editors*

September 2016
Advances in Neuroscience in Anesthesia and Critical Care
W. Andrew Kofke, *Editor*

RELATED INTEREST

Nursing Clinics of North America, March 2016 (Vol. 51, No. 1)
Pharmacology Updates
Jennifer Wilbeck, *Editor*
Available at: http://www.nursing.theclinics.com/

Foreword
Pharmacology

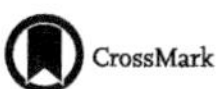

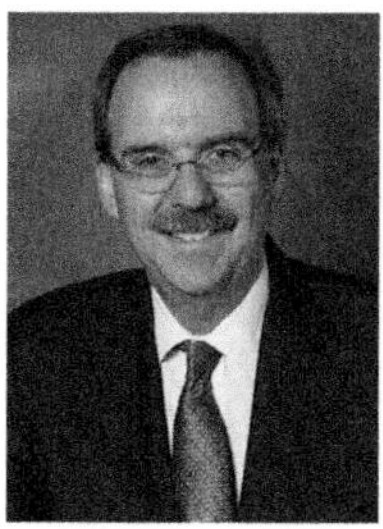

Lee A. Fleisher, MD, FACC
Consulting Editor

As anesthesiologists, we are the clinical pharmacologists of acute care medicine. We employ medications to induce anesthesia, relieve pain, and manipulate the cardiovascular and nervous system. There are also medications that are used in special populations, such as obstetrics and the geriatric population. In this issue, the authors have provided a more complete understanding of these medications and their effects in order for us to better manage our patients through the perioperative period.

This issue was proposed and edited by a leader in thought in this arena: Alan D. Kaye, MD, PhD, Professor and Chairman of the Department of Anesthesiology at LSU Health Sciences Center in New Orleans. He received two BS degrees and an MD degree from the University of Arizona. Dr Kaye completed his PhD in pharmacology in May 1997. He trained in Anesthesiology at Massachusetts General Hospital and Tulane University. He also completed a pain management fellowship at Texas Tech Health Sciences Center. He has authored or coauthored over 175 abstracts and 750 manuscripts and book chapters in the fields of pulmonary vascular pharmacology and anesthesiology and is on the FDA Advisory Board on Anesthetics and Analgesics. He has brought together a phenomenal group of authors to create this issue as well as a large group of additional articles online.

Lee A. Fleisher, MD, FACC
Perelman School of Medicine at
University of Pennsylvania
3400 Spruce Street, Dulles 680
Philadelphia, PA 19104, USA

E-mail address:
Lee.Fleisher@uphs.upenn.edu

Anesthesiology Clin 35 (2017) xvii
http://dx.doi.org/10.1016/j.anclin.2017.03.002
1932-2275/17/© 2017 Published by Elsevier Inc.

Preface

The Future of Pharmacology in Anesthesia Practice

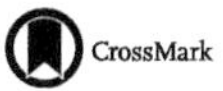

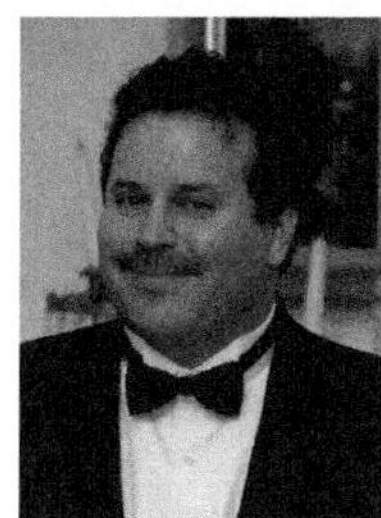

Alan D. Kaye, MD, PhD, DABA, DABPM, DABIPP
Editor

As a second year medical student, my oldest child, Aaron, recently started his pharmacology course at the Medical University of South Carolina in Charleston. Though the first lecture on pharmacokinetics left him terrorized, over time, he saw the wonders of understanding how drugs work in the human body. So much so, at present, he is considering a career as a future anesthesiologist.

This excites me because as he learned about the adrenergic system, I explained how my wife was placed on terbutaline, my favorite drug in the world, which relaxed her uterus, and gave my son and daughter, who is currently an undergraduate and premed student herself, safe passage into this world. In fact, who among us cannot appreciate the greatness of pharmacology in our lives?

Thinking back over my clinical career as an anesthesiologist, intensivist, and pain specialist, I have seen the wonders of pharmacology first hand and am delighted to share a very diverse group of articles focused on different drug considerations. Some of these topics are focused on subpopulations, including pediatrics, the obese, and geriatrics. For all of these varied patients, it is clear that there are very different pharmacokinetics and physiology in these groups, and I hope these reviews are meaningful for your practices.

There are focuses on different and important groups of drugs related to our field. Reviews in this issue include updates on novel anesthetics, opioid agents, local anesthetics, antiemetics, anticoagulants and their reversal, total parenteral nutrition, nonopioid intravenous or oral analgesics, uterotonic medications, pulmonary vascular mediating drugs, alpha 2 modulators, cardiovascular drugs, octreotide, nonsteroidal anti-inflammatory and steroid medications. In addition, there are interesting reviews on pharmacogenomics of pain and anesthesia, allowing us to look at our field in a different and futuristic manner.

Finally, we have included a special review as well on the basic pharmacology of oxycodone with a special emphasis on pharmacokinetic/pharmacodynamic properties. In

Anesthesiology Clin 35 (2017) xix–xx
http://dx.doi.org/10.1016/j.anclin.2017.03.001
1932-2275/17/© 2017 Published by Elsevier Inc.

addition, a special review is provided on the controversy regarding oxycodone-mediated or modulated effects for visceral pain via agonism, and the possible role or roles of peripheral opioid analgesia is discussed.

Our authors come from outstanding institutions from around the country, and I am especially thankful to Dr Lee Fleisher, Professor and Chairman of Anesthesiology at the University of Pennsylvania and my good friend, for giving me yet another opportunity to edit this series, and Dr Jonathan Jahr, a professor at UCLA and my longtime friend, for serving as a liaison and mentor on many of these review articles. I also want to thank the many members of my beloved LSU Department of Anesthesiology in New Orleans, who worked on a wide range of topics for this issue.

The future in anesthesiology is bright because of the development of newer and safer drugs and advancements in technology. We are living at a time where miracles happen in our operating rooms, in our intensive care units, and in pain management on a daily basis. Yet to come, we will have even more exciting opportunities to make a difference in the care of our patients with newer drugs and therapeutic options in the treatment of diseases and in the operating room. In this spirit, let us rededicate ourselves to our practices in medicine and find time always to have balance in our lives as we move forward to the future!

Alan D. Kaye, MD, PhD, DABA, DABPM, DABIPP
Department of Anesthesiology and Pharmacology
Anesthesiology Services
University Medical Center Hospital
Louisiana State University School of Medicine T6M5
1542 Tulane Avenue, Room 656
New Orleans, LA 70112, USA

E-mail address:
alankaye44@hotmail.com

Total Parenteral and Enteral Nutrition in the ICU

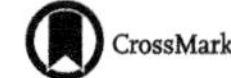

Evolving Concepts

Amir O. Elhassan, MD[a], Lien B. Tran, MD[a], Richard C. Clarke, MD[a], Sumit Singh, MD[b], Alan D. Kaye, MD, PhD, DABA, DABPM, DABIPP[a,*]

KEYWORDS

• Nutritional support • Enteral nutrition • ICU • Supplemental parenteral nutrition

KEY POINTS

- Appropriate nutrition in the hospital setting, particularly in critically ill patients, has long been tied to improving clinical outcomes.
- During critical illness, inflammatory mediators and cytokines lead to the creation of a catabolic state to facilitate the use of endogenous energy sources to meet increased energy demands. This process results in increasing the likelihood of overfeeding, making accurate nutritional support estimation and provision significant.
- Recognition of this significance has resulted in numerous work by the medical scientific community describing methods of calculation of energy requirements and use of appropriate routes, doses, timing, and adjuncts to nutritional support to complement treatment regimens in the critically ill patient.
- Although it is widely accepted that nutritional support via the enteral route has physiologic benefits, including maintenance of gut structural and functional integrity, digestive inadequacy in the acute phase of critical illness often favors parenteral nutrition, which in turn has been tied to infectious complications related to hyperalimentation and hyperglycemia.
- The scientific literature in the past 30 years reveals exponential advances in the understanding of molecular basis of nutritional support and evolution of clinical protocols aimed at treating artificial nutritional support as a therapeutic intervention, preventing loss of lean body mass and metabolic deterioration to improve clinical outcomes in the critically ill.

INTRODUCTION

Homeostasis in the critically ill patient is significantly disrupted related to a multitude of factors. Pathophysiologic aberrations, in combination with environmental, psychosocial, and nutritional stressors, contribute to this disruption. The mediators of the

[a] Department of Anesthesiology, Louisiana State University Health Sciences Center, 1542 Tulane Avenue, New Orleans, LA 70112, USA; [b] Department of Anesthesiology, David Geffen UCLA School of Medicine, 757 Westwood Plaza, Los Angeles, CA 90095, USA
* Corresponding author.
E-mail address: alankaye44@hotmail.com

Anesthesiology Clin 35 (2017) 181–190
http://dx.doi.org/10.1016/j.anclin.2017.01.004 anesthesiology.theclinics.com
1932-2275/17/

inflammatory component of critical illness often lead to altered energy consumption, which can result in depletion of energy stores. Timely delivery of appropriate nutritional support is, therefore, an integral part of the critically ill patient's care. Lack of sufficient enteral nutrition (EN) can cause a proinflammatory state, resulting in increased oxidative stress, multiorgan failure and a prolonged length of stay (LOS).[1–4] Moreover, early and appropriate enteral feeding can improve outcomes and decrease costs by improving LOS, namely by decreasing bacterial translocation across the gut, maintaining gut-associated lymphoid tissue (GALT) and preserving upper respiratory tract immunity.[1,2] On the other hand, supplemental parenteral nutrition (PN) allows for timely adequate feeding and plays a pivotal role in patients with intolerance to EN, provided that overfeeding is avoided by careful prescription based on energy expenditure measurement or precise estimation.[5] The dynamic metabolic and pathophysiologic changes in acute critical illness require that nutritional support be regarded as a form of pharmacotherapy aimed at improving clinical outcome.

This review article describes indications of nutritional support and discusses the current evidence-based guidelines on the estimation of energy demands as well as initiation and advancement of nutritional support. In addition, the current investigation reviews adjunctive therapy and drug interactions related to artificial nutritional support as well as specific indications of PN. Finally, a comparison of EN and PN based on outcome studies focusing on the ICU setting is discussed.

INITIATION AND ADVANCEMENT OF NUTRITIONAL SUPPORT

Benefits of Early Enteral Nutrition

EN has been found beneficial within the first 24 hours to 48 hours in the critically ill patient who is unable to maintain volitional intake.[2] Providing EN maintains gut integrity, stress modulation, systemic immune response, and attenuation of disease severity. After a major insult or injury, gut permeability increases from the loss of functional integrity. This event is time dependent and can result in increased bacterial challenge (engagement of GALT with enteric organisms), risk for systemic infection, and greater likelihood of multiple-organ dysfunction syndrome. As disease severity worsens, increases in gut permeability are amplified, and the enteral route of feeding is more likely to cause a greater impact on outcome parameters of infection, organ failure, and hospital LOS.[2]

Estimating Energy Needs

The gold standard for estimating energy needs of the critically ill patient remains indirect calorimetry (IC). The American Society of Parenteral and Enteral Nutrition (ASPEN) guidelines recommend use of IC when available and in the absence of other variables that can affect accuracy of measurement.[2] Although superior to other methods discussed later, the practicality of IC in the ICU is limited in most hospitals due to availability and cost. Factors that can affect the accuracy of IC are numerous and include the presence of air leaks or chest tubes, use of supplemental oxygen and mechanical ventilation settings, continuous renal replacement therapy, anesthesia, and excessive patient movement.[6] Clinicians are, therefore, obliged to use a surrogate for calculating estimated energy requirement.

There are more than 200 equations developed for estimation of energy needs in the critically ill. No single equation has emerged as the most accurate in the ICU setting. The Academy of Nutrition and Dietetics recommends using the Penn State University 2003 equation[2,7] or the Penn State University 2010 equation for obese patients over the age of 65.[2,8] The ASPEN position in this matter is that equations derived from testing hospital patients (Penn State, Ireton-Jones, and Swinamer equations) are no more accurate than equations derived from testing normal volunteers (Harris-Benedict and Mifflin–St Jeor equations).[9] The poor accuracy of predictive equations is related to many nonstatic variables affecting energy expenditure in the critically ill patient, such as weight, medications, treatments, and body temperature. The only advantage of using weight-based equations over other predictive equations is simplicity.[2] The most simplistic equation in clinical use is an estimation of 25 kcal/kg/d to 30 kcal/kg/d. Prevention of underfeeding and overfeeding can be achieved by a continuous reevaluation of energy expenditure, more than once per week, and strategies to optimize energy and protein intake should be used.[2]

Adequate protein supplementation is the most important element of nutritional support in the critical care setting, affecting immune function, wound healing, and lean body mass maintenance. Weight-based equations estimate 1.2 g/kg to 2.0 g/kg actual body weight/d as the target protein amount, whereas in the obese population, 2.0 g/kg to 2.5 g/kg ideal body weight/d is required. Serum protein markers, such as albumin, prealbumin, transferrin, and C-reactive protein, are not validated for determining adequacy of protein provision and should not be used in the critical care setting in this manner.[2,10–12]

Initiation and Maintenance

For critically ill patients who are unable to maintain volitional intake, initiation of EN support should begin within 24 hours to 48 hours of ICU admission. In the majority of critically ill patients, it is more practical and safe to use EN as opposed to PN.[2] Trophic feeds at a rate of 10 mL/h to 20 mL/h may be sufficient to prevent mucosal atrophy and maintain gut integrity and are recommended as an acceptable start rate. EN should then be advanced to goal rate by 10 mL/h to 20 mL/h every 8 hours to 12 hours as tolerated.[12] There are no EN initiation and advancement protocols studied and proved associated with better outcomes. Expert opinion generally advises to advance trophic EN as tolerated.

Gastrointestinal intolerance is usually defined by clinical symptoms, such as complaints of discomfort, as well as by clinical signs, such as abdominal distention, diarrhea, absence of flatus, and increases in nasograstic output and gastric residual volume (GRV). McClave and colleagues[13] reported that more than 97% of nurses surveyed assessed intolerance solely by measuring GRVs (the most frequently cited threshold levels for interrupting EN listed as 200 mL and 250 mL). According to the ASPEN guidelines, for those ICUs where GRVs are still used, holding EN for GRVs less than 500 mL in the absence of other signs of intolerance should be avoided. This is due to lack of sufficient data that GRVs correlate well with the incidence of pneumonia, aspiration, or regurgitation. In a prospective study of 206 critically ill patients, McClave and colleagues[13] showed that GRVs (over a range of 150–400 mL) were shown to be a poor monitor for aspiration, with a very low sensitivity of 1.5% to 4.1%, a positive predictive value of 18.2% to 25%, and a negative predictive value of 77.1% to 77.4%. Furthermore, multiple trials have shown that eliminating the use of GRV to assess EN improves delivery of EN without jeopardizing patient safety.[14–16] Using other means of assessment of gastrointestinal intolerance, discussed previously, along with abdominal radiographs is sufficient to provide adequate EN while monitoring risks of aspiration and pneumonia. Because most ICUs still use GRV, it is recommended to assess aspiration prophylaxis and causality of possible intolerance at GRV 200 mL to 500 mL but not complete cessation of EN at GRV less than 500 mL because this increases the risk of underfeeding.

For short-term enteral feeding, an orogastric or nasogastric route is preferred, related to ease of placement. For long-term need (more than 4 weeks), placement of a long-term feeding device, such as gastrostomy or jejunostomy tube, should be considered.[12] Postpyloric enteral device placement is recommended for patients with history of gastric feeds intolerance or those with a known history or high risk of aspiration.[2] Changing the level of infusion of EN from the stomach to the small bowel has been shown to reduce the incidence of regurgitation, aspiration, and pneumonia.[17,18]

When to Use Parenteral Nutrition

Given the risks and clinical outcomes attributed to PN, discussed previously, careful consideration should be used when considering PN for critically ill patients. Two factors should be considered when making this decision: nutrition risk and adequacy of EN in meeting energy and protein goals.[2] The Nutrition Risk Screening (NRS 2002) and the Nutrition Risk in the Critically Ill (NUTRIC) tools are widely used for nutrition risk assessment and recognized by ASPEN for that purpose.

- Low nutrition risk patients: for patients determined to be at low nutrition risk (eg, NRS 2002 $\leq$3 or NUTRIC score $\leq$5), exclusive PN be withheld over the first 7 days after ICU admission if patients cannot maintain volitional intake and if early EN is not feasible.
- High nutrition risk patients: for ICU patients determined to be at high nutrition risk (eg, NRS 2002 $\geq$5 or NUTRIC score $\geq$5) or severely malnourished, when EN is not feasible, exclusive PN should be begun as soon as possible after ICU admission.
- Inadequate EN: whether at high or low nutrition risk, PN supplementation of EN should be started in patients in whom greater than 60% of estimated energy and protein requirement cannot be met by EN alone after 7 days to 10 days. Supplemental PN prior to this 7-day to 10-day period in critically ill patients on some EN does not improve outcomes and may be detrimental.[2]

ADJUNCTIVE THERAPY

Fiber

The addition of fiber supplementation in the form of fermentable soluble fiber additive, such as fructooligossaccharides (FOS) and inulin, should be considered for use in all hemodynamically stable critically ill patients. The addition of 10 g to 20 g of a fermentable soluble fiber supplement in divided doses over 24 hours as an adjunctive therapy should be considered particularly if there is evidence of diarrhea.[2]

FOS are a group of insoluble carbohydrates fermented in the colon into short-chain fatty acids. The trophic effect of short-chain fatty acids on the colonocyte stimulates the uptake of water and electrolytes, thereby benefiting patients with diarrhea.[19] Prebiotics (eg, inulin and FOS) stimulate the growth of commensal microbiota and promote bowel health.[2] Patients with feeding intolerance have been shown to have significantly lower amounts of beneficial commensal anaerobes and higher amounts of staphylococcus in stool analysis.[20]

Probiotics

Probiotics are viable microorganisms that, when ingested in adequate amounts, can be beneficial for health (World Health Organization definition). Multiple factors in the ICU settings affect the presence and function of commensal microorganisms, including wide-spectrum antibiotic use. Nevertheless, no consistent benefit has been shown in the general population to warrant their prescription for the general ICU population. Although they have been shown beneficial in decreasing ventilator-associated pneumonia and general infections,[21] they are only recommended in patient populations in whom randomized controlled trials have shown a clear benefit.[2]

Antioxidants and Trace Minerals

Provision of antioxidant vitamins, including vitamins E and C, and trace minerals, including selenium, zinc, and copper, may improve outcome in burns, trauma, and critical illness requiring mechanical ventilation.[22,23] Issues of administration, such as dosage, frequency, and route of administration, have not been well established. In addition, renal dysfunction should be closely considered when prescribing vitamins and trace elements to prevent toxicity.

Glutamine, Arginine, Eicosapentaenoic Acid, Docosahexaenoic Acid, and Nucleic Acid

Reducing rates of infection and decreased LOS and duration of mechanical ventilation have been proposed as potential benefits of using immune-modulating enteral formulations, such as glutamine, arginine, eicosapentaenoic acid (EPA), docosahexaenoic acid (DHA), and nucleic acids in the ICU settings. Glutamine is a key substrate for gluconeogenesis and is an important fuel for rapid turnover cells, such as the small intestine epithelium and immune cells, including lymphocytes and macrophages.[24,25] Additionally, it is involved in the regulation of T-cell proliferation, interleukin 2 production, and B-cell differentiation, as well as having a role in phagocytosis and superoxide production.[25] The ASPEN guidelines, however, do not recommend routine addition of immune-modulating enteral supplements in the medical ICU setting due to lack of significant and consistent outcome improvement seen in aggregation of available randomized controlled trials.[2] Many commercially available enteral feeds do, however, contain glutamine, which address this issue in most patients. In the surgical ICU setting, the ASPEN guidelines, however, recommend arginine containing immune-modulating formulations or EPA/DHA supplement with standard enteral formula in patients with traumatic brain injury and postoperative surgical patients.[2]

DRUG INTERACTIONS

Drug interactions of EN/PN with intravenous (IV) or enteral medications is a wide and complex topic. To reduce costs, IV medications are switched to the enteral route whenever possible in the ICU. This is a common and acceptable practice; however, it increases the risk of unreliable delivery due to EN effect on absorption and drug interaction with feeding tube material or EN formula.[26] Some general principles in practice to reduce these effects are as follows:[1]

- Feeding catheter tip location: depending on the medication formulation, an alkaline or acidic medium may be required for absorption. Use of gastric, duodenal, or jejunal tube for delivery should be considered.[26]
- Flushing of EN catheter: flushing of EN catheter should be performed before and after medication administration with 15 mL of water; similarly, 15 mL flush should be used between administration of different enteral drugs.[12]
- Formulation consistency: a liquid formulation or an elixir is the preferred form for administration through enteral catheters. This should be diluted with 30 mL of water before administration. Medications should never be mixed with EN formula.[12] Solid medications should be crushed into a powder and mixed with water to form a slurry before administration; gelatin capsules can be aspirated and should be dissolved in water prior to administration.[27]
- Prevention of catheter occlusion: gastric access is usually the preferred route of medication administration because those catheters have a larger lumen and are

less likely to get blocked. Smaller catheters (eg, jejunostomy tubes) should only be used for liquid formulations to prevent occlusion.

Table 1 lists some examples of enteral drug formulations' known interactions with EN or EN catheters. It is advised for such drugs that EN is held 1 hour before and 1 hour after administration. When appropriate, serum drug levels (eg, theophylline and phenytoin) should be monitored to ensure adequate delivery. Serum markers of drug effect (eg, prothrombin time for warfarin and thyroid-stimulating hormone levels for levothyroxine) can also be used to ensure adequate delivery and dosing adjustments can be made appropriately.

Although pure inotropes, such as milrinone and dobutamine, improve cardiac output and increase gut perfusion, administration of vasopressors in hemodynamically stable patients receiving EN could result in bowel ischemia and EN intolerance.[1,32,33] This risk does not pose a contraindication to EN; this subset of patients (hemodynamically unstable on multiple vasopressors) may benefit the most from early EN therapy. Early EN and careful advancement should be considered in these patients, and, if not well tolerated, complete or supplemental PN should be considered.

Propofol does not directly interact with EN but can increase the risk of overfeeding by providing additional kilocalories. Due to its formulation as a lipid solution containing 1.1 kcal/mL, propofol administered at high rates continuously can provide a significant amount of lipid kilocalories. Daily calorie intake from propofol should be monitored and nutritional support manipulated accordingly to prevent overfeeding.

SIDE EFFECTS

Using a nutritional support team, including physicians, registered dieticians, pharmacists, and registered nurses, improves the safety and side-effect profile of nutrition

Table 1
Examples of common enteral drug formulations' interaction with enteral nutrition

Enteral Drug	Enteral Nutrition Interaction
Penicillin V	Bioavailability varies 30%–80% with concomitant administration of food.[1]
Proton pump inhibitors	Commonly available as enteric-coated delayed-release granules or tablets.[28] Mixing delayed-release capsules (omeprazole and lansoprazole) with acidic diluents (apple or orange juice) helps to keep the granules intact until they reach the duodenum. Because there is a potential for occlusion by clumping of granules, especially through small-bore feeding tubes, another method of administration includes alkaline suspensions made by dissolving granules in a solution of 8.4% sodium bicarbonate.[26]
Theophylline	A >30% decrease of theophylline level has been reported with enteral feeding.[29]
Levothyroxine sodium	May bind with EN feeding tubes, resulting in decreased drug efficacy.[30]
Warfarin	Binding of warfarin with proteins in the EN can reduce bioavailability and decrease the anticoagulant effect.[31]
Carbamazepine	Adherence of carbamazepine to the walls of polyvinyl chloride can result inadequate drug delivery.[26]
Phenytoin	Absorption of phenytoin may be reduced by 70% when administered concurrently with EN; impaired absorption includes adherence to the tube itself and binding to proteins and calcium salts.[1,26]

support. Common side effects of EN and PN, recommended methods of prevention, treatment recommendations, and a brief summary of available data comparing the side effects of PN and EN are discussed.

Side Effects of Enteral Nutrition

Most studies investigating immune-modulating EN have shown benefit in critically ill patients.[1,17] ASPEN currently recommends use of immune-modulating EN, including arginine, in several critically ill patient populations, such as medical ICU patients, severe trauma, traumatic brain injury, and postoperative patients but recommends against their use in severe sepsis. Theoretically, arginine metabolism can result in an increase in nitric oxide production, causing hemodynamic instability in severe sepsis.[2,17] There are, however, several studies that should improve outcomes in these patients with arginine containing immune-modulating EN support.[2,17]

In patients with renal failure, the metabolism of the high protein content of immune-modulating EN, in addition to that of arginine and glutamine, may increase blood urea nitrogen and complicate therapy.[1,17] Low protein, or renal formula, is preferred in these patients.

EN delivered into the stomach may increase the risk of esophageal reflux. Nasojejunal tubes may be preferable in patients with a known risk of aspiration or with a history of gastric feeds intolerance.[2,17,18]At this time, there is insufficient evidence to support routine placement of jejunal tubes over gastric tubes in critically ill patients.[1,34]

Side Effects of Parenteral Nutrition

Hyperglycemia is the most common complication associated with PN. IV dextrose causes a more pronounced hyperglycemia than expected from an equal amount administered enterically. This is caused by IV dextrose bypassing the enteroinsular axis.[35] To prevent hyperglycemia, PN should be initiated and advanced slowly while blood glucose is closely monitored and insulin administration carefully titrated. In addition, ASPEN recommends that daily carbohydrate administration rate should not exceed 4 mg/kg/min to 5 mg/kg/min for critically ill and diabetic patients.[36]

IV fat emulsion (IVFE) included in PN can cause hypertriglyceridemia when PN is administered rapidly. Hyperlipidemia increases the risk of pancreatitis and may worsen immune function.[36] Patients who develop hyperlipidemia may require cyclic IVFE infusion with 12-hour to 24-hour interruptions and minimal IVFE volume. Patients with soy and egg allergy may not tolerate IVFE because it contains an egg phospholipid emulsifier and trace soy proteins. IVFE should be initiated and advanced slowly to monitor tolerance and avoided in those with soy or egg allergies.

Perhaps the most severe side effect of PN is PN-associated liver disease (PNALD), which is a spectrum of issues, including steatosis, cholestasis, and gallstones, and may progress to cirrhosis if not managed appropriately.[37] The etiology of PNALD is complex, including hepatotoxic effects of PN, inappropriate PN management leading to overfeeding, and lack of enteral stimulation. Management of PNALD includes prevention of carbohydrate and/or lipid overfeeding, using EN or an oral diet to stimulate bile flow when possible, and cycling PN off for 8 hours to 10 hours a day. Clinicians should also consider other underlying causes, including small bowel bacterial overgrowth (which may be related to nutrition therapy), hepatotoxic medications, and infection as causes of hepatic dysfunction.[37]

PN increases risk of all infections, including central line infections. Patients receiving PN therapy have a higher prevalence of pneumonia and intra-abdominal abscess, in addition to line sepsis.[37] There is also increased risk of mortality from line infections.[37] The risk of infection can be decreased with the use of appropriate dedicated ports only, proper catheter placement and care, and delaying initiation of PN or holding PN until infections have been adequately treated.[1] If line sepsis is suspected, the central venous catheter should be removed and should not be replaced until the infection has been adequately treated.

Comparison of Enteral Nutrition and Parenteral Nutrition Side Effects

An updated meta-analysis by Elke and colleagues[38] on 18 randomized controlled trials with a total of 3347 critically ill adult patients reviews the effect of the route of nutrition (EN vs PN) on clinical outcomes. Overall, there was no difference in mortality between the 2 routes of nutrition. EN compared with PN led to a significant reduction in the number of infectious complications and ICU LOS whereas no significant effect was found with respect to hospital LOS and mechanical ventilation. The positive treatment effect of EN on infectious morbidity and ICU LOS may be attributed, however, to differences in caloric intake between study groups. Furthermore, funnel plot analysis revealed evidence for significant publication bias for the trials reporting on infectious complications.[38]

SUMMARY

The implications of artificial nutrition, including EN and PN, exceeds simple provision of nutrients. In the critically ill population, nutrition support is an integral part of the care plan and may affect patient outcomes, cost, and LOS. A team approach to nutritional support composed of trained clinicians improves its safety profile and clinical benefit and is highly recommended. Close monitoring of the effects of nutritional support by a clinical team and continuous modification of the type and contents of nutritional support are preferred to ensure the best medical and nutritional outcome in the critically ill patient population.

REFERENCES

1. Redgate J, Singh S. Enteral and Parenteral Nutrition. In: Kay AD, Kay AM, Urman RD, editors. Essentials of Pharmacology for Anesthesia, Pain Medicine, and Critical Care. New York: Springer Science + Business Media; 2015. p. 661–75.
2. McClave SA, Taylor BE, Martindale RG, et al. Guidelines for the provision and assessment of nutrition support therapy in the adult critically ill patient: Society of Critical Care Medicine (SCCM) and American Society for Parenteral and Enteral Nutrition (A.S.P.E.N.). JPEN J Parenter Enteral Nutr 2016;40(2):159–211.
3. Bengmark S. Gut microenvironment and immune function. Curr Opin Clin Nutr Metab 1999;2(1):84–5.
4. Carrico CJ. The elusive pathophysiology of the multiple organ failure syndrome. Ann Surg 1993;218(2):109–10.
5. Oshima T, Heidegger CP, Pichard C. Supplemental parenteral nutrition is the key to prevent energy deficits in critically ill patients. Nutr Clin Pract 2016;31(4): 432–7.
6. Schlein KM, Coulter SP. Best practices for determining resting energyexpenditure in critically ill adults. Nutr Clin Pract 2014;29(1):44–55.
7. Academy of Nutrition and Dietetics Evidence Analysis Library. If indirect calorimetry is unavailable or impractical, what is the best way to estimate resting metabolic rate (RMR) in non-obese adult critically ill patients? Academy of Nutrition and Dietetics. Available at: http://andevidencelibrary.com/conclusion.cfm?conclusion_statement_id=251361. Accessed March 6, 2013.

8. Academy of Nutrition and Dietetics Evidence Analysis Library. If indirect calorimetry is unavailable or impractical, what is the best way to estimate resting metabolic rate (RMR) in obese adult critically ill patients? Academy of Nutrition and Dietetics. Available at: http://andevidencelibrary.com/conclusion.cfm?conclusion_statement_id=251240. Accessed March 6, 2013.
9. Boullata J, Williams J, Cottrell F, et al. Accurate determination of energy needs in hospitalized patients. J Am Diet Assoc 2007;107(3):393–401.
10. Davis CJ, Sowa D, Keim KS, et al. The use of prealbumin and C-reactive protein for monitoring nutrition support in adult patients receiving enteral nutrition in an urban medical center. JPEN J Parenter Enteral Nutr 2012;36(2):197–204.
11. Stroud M. Protein and the critically ill; do we know what to give? Proc Nutr Soc 2007;66(3):378–83.
12. Lee JL, Oh ES, Lee RW, et al. Serum albumin and prealbumin and calorically restricted, Nondiseased individuals: a systematic review. Am J Med 2015; 128(9). 1023.e1-e22.
13. McClave SA, Lukan JK, Stefater JA, et al. Poor validity of residual volumes as a marker for risk of aspiration in critically ill patients. Crit Care Med 2005;33(2): 324–30.
14. Powell KS, Marcuard SP, Farrior ES, et al. Aspirating gastric residuals causes occlusion of small-bore feeding tubes. JPEN J Parenter Enteral Nutr 1993;17(3): 243–6.
15. Poulard F, Dimet J, Martin-Lefevre L, et al. Impact of not measuring residual gastric volume in mechanically ventilated patients receiving early enteral feeding: a prospective before-after study. JPEN J Parenter Enteral Nutr 2010;34(2): 125–30.
16. Reignier J, Mercier E, Le Gouge A, et al. Effect of not monitoring residual gastric volume on risk of ventilator-associated pneumonia in adults receiving mechanical ventilation and early enteral feeding: a randomized controlled trial. JAMA 2013; 309(3):249–56.
17. Heyland DK, Drover JW, MacDonald S, et al. Effect of postpyloric feeding on gastroesophageal regurgitation and pulmonary microaspiration: results of a randomized controlled trial. Crit Care Med 2001;29(8):1495–501.
18. Lien HC, Chang CS, Chen GH. Can percutaneous endoscopic jejunostomy prevent gastroesophageal reflux in patients with preexisting esophagitis? Am J Gastroenterol 2000;95(12):3439–43.
19. Kato Y, Nakao M, Iwasa M, et al. Soluble fiber improves management of diarrhea in elderly patients receiving enteral nutrition. Food Nutr Sci 2012;3:1547–52.
20. Shimizu K, Ogura H, Asahara T, et al. Gastrointestinal dysmotility is associated with altered gut flora and septic mortality in patients with severe systemic inflammatory response syndrome: a preliminary study. Neurogastroenterol Motil 2011; 23(4):330–5, e157.
21. Morrow LE, Kollef MH, Casale TB. Probiotic prophylaxis of ventilator associated pneumonia: a blinded, randomized, controlled trial. Am J Respir Crit Care Med 2010;182(8):1058–64.
22. Berger MM, Spertini F, Shenkin A, et al. Trace element supplementation modulates pulmonary infection rates after major burns: a double-blind, placebo-controlled trial. Am J Clin Nutr 1998;68(2):365–71.
23. Nathens AB, Neff MJ, Jurkovich GJ, et al. Randomized, prospective trial of antioxidant supplementation in critically ill surgical patients. Ann Surg 2002;236(6): 814–22.

24. Worthington ML, Cresci G. Immune-modulationg formulas: who wins the meta-analysis race? Nutr Clin Pract 2011;26(6):650–5.
25. Jayarajan S, Daly SM. The relationship of nutrients, routes of delivery, and immunocompetence. Surg Clin North Am 2011;91(4):737–53.
26. Williams NT. Medication administration through enteral feeding tubes. Am J Health Syst Pharm 2008;65(24):2347–57.
27. Belknap DC, Seifert CF, Petermann M. Administration of medications through enteral feeding catheters. Am J Crit Care 1997;6:382–92.
28. Howden CW. Review article: immediate-release proton-pump inhibitor therapy–potential advantages. Aliment Pharmacol Ther 2005;22(Suppl 3):25–30.
29. Gal P, Layson R. Interference with oral theophylline absorption by continuous nasogastric feedings. Ther Drug Monit 1986;8:421–3.
30. Smyrniotis V, Vaos N, Arkadopoulos N, et al. Severe hypothryoidism in patients dependent on prolonged thyroxine infusion through a jejunostomy. Clin Nutr 2000;19(1):65–7.
31. Dickerson RN, Garmon WM, Kuhl DA, et al. Vitamin K-independent warfarin resistance after concurrent administration of warfarin and continuous enteral nutrition. Pharmacotherapy 2008;28:308–13.
32. Khalid I, Doshi P, DiGiovine B. Early enteral nutrition and outcome of critically ill patients treated with vasopressors and mechanical ventilation. Am J Crit Care 2010;19(3):261–8.
33. Lowrey TS, Dunlap AW, Brown RO, et al. Pharmacologic influence on nutrition support therapy: use of propofol in a patient receiving combined enteral and parenteral nutrition support. Nutr Clin Pract 1996;11(4):147–9.
34. Casaer MP, Mesotten D, Hermans G, et al. Early versus late parenteral nutrition in critically ill adults. N Engl J Med 2011;365(6):506–17.
35. Buchman AL, Ament ME. Comparative hypersensitivity in intravenous lipid emulsions. JPEN J Parenter Enteral Nutr 1991;15(3):345–6.
36. Mirtallo J, Canada T, Johnson D, et al. Safe practices for parenteral nutrition. JPEN J Parenter Enteral Nutr 2004;28(6):S39–70.
37. Kudsk KA, Croce MA, Fabian TC, et al. Enteral versus parenteral feeding: effects on septic morbidity after blunt and penetrating abdominal trauma. Ann Surg 1992;215:503–11.
38. Elke G, van Zanten AR, Lemieux M, et al. Enteral versus parenteral nutrition incritically ill patients: an updated systematic review and meta-analysis of randomized controlled trials. Crit Care 2016;20:117.

Anticoagulant Reversal and Anesthetic Considerations

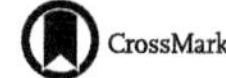

Joseph Meltzer, MD[a], Joseph R. Guenzer, MD[b,*]

KEYWORDS

- Laboratory monitoring • Prothrombin complex concentrates
- Specific reversal agents • Factor Xa inhibitors • Direct thrombin inhibitors

KEY POINTS

- Bleeding complications are a common concern with the use of anticoagulant agents. In many situations, reversing of neutralizing their effects may be warranted.
- Prothrombin complex concentrate (PCC) replaces coagulation factors lowered by warfarin, as does fresh frozen plasma (FFP), but in a more concentrated form.
- Protamine negates the effect of heparin and combines chemically with heparin molecules to form an inactive salt. It also partially reverses the effects of low-molecular-weight heparin (LMWH).
- Recombinant activated factor VII is a nonspecific procoagulant that activates the extrinsic clotting pathway resulting in thrombin generation but does not directly neutralize the activity of any of the new oral anticoagulants.
- Dabigatran etexilate is an oral direct thrombin inhibitor (DTI) that can be reversed with both PCC and idarucizumab.
- Rivaroxaban, apixaban, and edoxaban are all oral factor Xa inhibitors that can be reversed with PCC, andexanet alfa, and cirapirantag.

INTRODUCTION

Anticoagulants are an important part of the treatment of many disease processes, including atrial fibrillation,[1] venous thromboembolism (VTE),[2] arterial thromboembolism (ATE),[3] and intrinsic hypercoagulable states. They also play a key role in various surgical procedures, such as cardiac and vascular surgeries, as well as percutaneous catheter-based interventions. These agents cause an appreciable increase, however, in the risk of spontaneous hemorrhage[4] and a decrement in hemostasis, as seen in

[a] Department of Anesthesiology, David Geffen School of Medicine, University of California, Los Angeles, Los Angeles, CA 90095, USA; [b] Department of Anesthesiology, University of Utah Medical School, 30 North 1900 East, Room 3C444, Salt Lake City, UT 84132-2501, USA
* Corresponding author.
E-mail address: Joseph.Guenzer@hsc.utah.edu

Anesthesiology Clin 35 (2017) 191–205
http://dx.doi.org/10.1016/j.anclin.2017.01.005
1932-2275/17/Published by Elsevier Inc.
anesthesiology.theclinics.com

higher transfusion requirements during surgery.[5] Understanding the pharmacokinetics and clinical effect of these agents as well as effective strategies for anticoagulant reversal is key for effective and safe provision of anesthesia, especially in emergencies.

AVAILABLE AGENTS

A wide variety of anticoagulant agents are available (**Table 1**). These agents have various mechanisms of action (**Figure 1**), duration of effect, and method of reversal.

HEPARINS

Heparins are naturally occurring glycosaminoglycans.[19] Their native function is at this time unproved. Heparins are commonly used for both treatment and prevention of thrombosis due to their ability to bind antithrombin III (ATIII) and thereby inhibit function of factor Xa and thrombin (factor IIa) as well as factors IXa, XIa, and XIIa.[20] Thrombin inhibition requires the heparin molecule to simultaneously bind ATIII and thrombin. LMWHs are too small to bind ATIII and thrombin simultaneously and are far more specific for inhibition of Xa.[19]

Heparins are typically isolated from bovine or porcine sources. It is thought that porcine heparins are safer due to a lower risk of heparin-induced thrombocytopenia (HIT), an immune-mediated disorder.[21] Unfractionated heparin is a mix of heparins of varying molecular weights, ranging in size from 3000 Da to 30,000 Da, with the molecule having an average mass of 15,000 Da.[19] Heparin activity is classically monitored by activated partial thromboplastin time (aPTT), although the evidence for this is poor and therapeutic ranges must be institution specific due to variability in test reagents and protocols.[22]

LMWHs, such as enoxaparin, are purified to select out smaller molecules, typically of 4000 Da to 9000 Da. These smaller molecules are more specific for Xa inhibition,[23] have more reliable pharmacokinetics,[24] and carry a lower risk of HIT.[25] Fondaparinux is a synthetic pentasaccharide that preserves the ATIII-binding domain of heparin, preserving the active site.[26] Like LMWH, fondaparinux has more predictable kinetics and is more selective for activity against factor Xa. Routine monitoring of LMWHs is not recommended. If necessary, anti-Xa activity should be assayed.

Indications

Heparin is indicated for a wide variety of conditions. Subcutaneous heparin, either unfractionated or LMWH, is frequently administered to hospitalized patients for the prevention of VTE.[2] Intravenous unfractionated heparin, most commonly as a continuous infusion, and subcutaneous LMWH are indicated for the treatment of VTE,[2] ATE,[3] and acute myocardial infarction. Bolus doses of unfractionated heparin are commonly given during cardiac and vascular surgeries as well as catheter-based interventions. Additionally, patients with mechanical prosthetic valves, ventricular assist devices (VADs), and on extracorporeal membrane oxygenation (ECMO) support must be maintained on systemic anticoagulation at all times for prevention of device thrombosis, and heparin is often used during bridging or hospitalization.[27]

Kinetics

Unfractionated heparin can be given either intravenously or subcutaneously. Intravenous heparin reaches peak effect within 3 minutes and has an elimination half-life of 1 hour to 1.5 hours.[28] Subcutaneous unfractionated heparin reaches peak effect

Table 1
Summary of anticoagulant agents available in the United States

Agent	Mechanism	Route	T Peak	Half-life	Route of Elimination	Reversal
Unfractionated heparin[6]	Binds ATIII, neutralizes thrombin, Xa	IV, SQ	IV: 1–3 min SQ: 2–4 h	IV: 1–1.5 h SQ: 1.5 h	Hepatic, endothelial metabolism	Protamine, cirapirantag
Enoxaparin[7]	Neutralizes Xa via ATIII	SQ	3–5 h	7 h	Hepatic depolymerization, renal excretion	Protamine, cirapirantag
Fondaparinux[8]	Neutralizes Xa via ATIII	SQ	3 h	17–21 h	77% renal	cirapirantag
VKAs (warfarin)[9]	Block hepatic synthesis of vitamin K dependent factors	Oral	4 h	Variable	Extensive hepatic metabolism, renal excretion	Vitamin K, FFP, PCC
Lepirudin[10]	Directly blocks thrombin activity	IV	Immediate	1 h	Renal clearance	None
Desirudin[11]	Directly blocks thrombin activity	SQ	N/A	2 h	Renal clearance	None
Bivalirudin[12]	Directly blocks thrombin activity	IV	Immediate	25 min	Renal metabolism, plasma proteolysis	None
Argatroban[13]	Directly blocks thrombin activity	IV	30 min	30–51 min, up to 180 min in liver failure	Hepatic hydroxylation and aromatization	None
Dabigatran etexilate[14,15]	Directly blocks thrombin activity, prodrug of dabigatran	Oral	2 h	8–13 h	Hepatic glucuronidation, renal clearance	Idarucizumab
Rivaroxaban[16]	Directly blocks Xa activity	Oral	2–4 h	5–11 h	CYP3A4, renal clearance	Andexanet alfa, cirapirantag
Apixaban[17]	Directly blocks Xa activity	Oral	3–4 h	6–15 h	CYP3A4, renal clearance	Andexanet alfa, cirapirantag
Edoxaban[18]	Directly blocks Xa activity	Oral	1–2 h	10–14 h	Renal and biliary clearance	Andexanet alfa, cirapirantag

Abbreviations: IV, intravenous; SQ, subcutaneous.

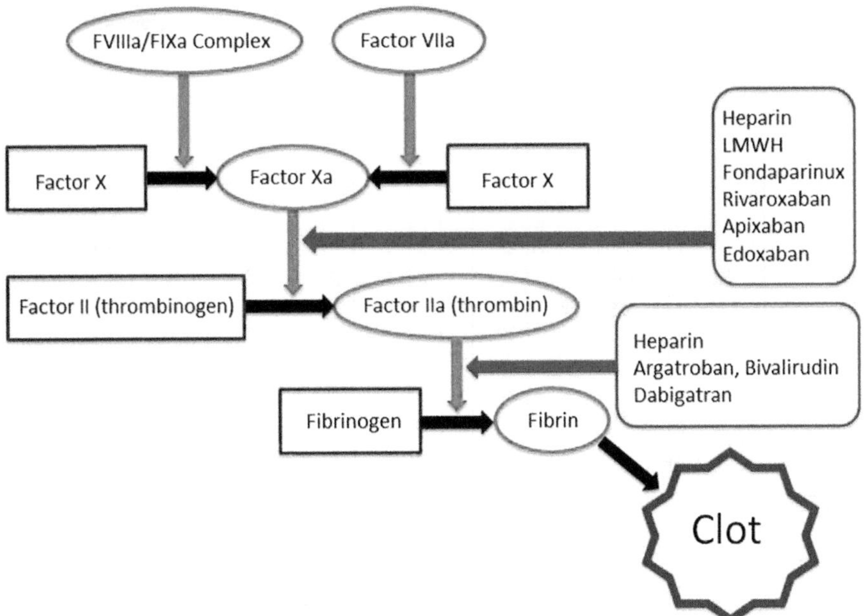

Fig. 1. The common pathway of the coagulation cascade. Blue: inactive clotting factors. Green: activated clotting factors. Red: anticoagulants, with the red arrows indicating mechanism of action (ie, activated clotting factor, which is antagonized). FVIIIa/FIXa Complex, Factor VIIIa/Factor IXa Complex.

within 2 hours to 4 hours and has an elimination half-life of 1.5 hours. Heparin is metabolized by the liver via N-desulfation.[29] The reticuloendothelial system and macrophage phagocytosis also contribute to metabolism. Unfractionated heparin is not dialyzable.

Enoxaparin is given subcutaneously and is predictably absorbed with peak effect observed in 3 hours to 5 hours.[24] Bioavailability is 90% after subcutaneous administration. Protein and endothelial binding is limited, thereby making the kinetics more predictable. Enoxaparin is depolymerized by the liver and excreted by the kidneys. Renal failure contributes to prolonged elimination. Enoxaparin is poorly dialyzable.

Fondaparinux is given subcutaneously and is predictably absorbed with peak effect observed in 2 hours to 3 hours. Fondaparinux is more than 75% cleared by kidneys with an elimination half-life of 17 hours to 21 hours. Approximately 20% of systemic fondaparinux can be cleared by hemodialysis.[30]

Reversal

Although its pharmacokinetics are unpredictable, a main advantage of unfractionated heparin compared with LMWHs is the ease of reversal. Protamine rapidly and reliably reverses heparin by aPTT[31]; 1 mg of protamine typically reverses 100 U of heparin. Because of the kinetics of heparin during continuous infusion, only heparin given during the past 2 hours to 3 hours needs to be considered for reversal. Protamine is not without its own adverse effects.[32] Rapid administration may cause bradycardia, hypotension, and pulmonary hypotension, so slow administration is preferred. Additionally, protamine is immunogenic. Patients on maintenance NPH insulin, men who have had a vasectomy, and patients with known fish sensitivity (protamine is isolated from fish sperm) may be at increased risk of anaphylactic reactions.[32] No other reversal agents are available at this time.

Protamine only incompletely reverse the anticoagulant effect of LMWHs[33] and does not seem to have any effect on fondaparinux. No prospective data exist, however, on the clinical implications of protamine reversal of LMWHs. Because no other proved reversal agents exist, the American College of Chest Physicians recommends that protamine be given to hemorrhaging patients who received LMWH within the last 8 hours.[34] Andexanet alfa, an inactivated factor Xa analog designed for the reversal of direct Xa inhibitors (discussed later), seems to have some ability to reverse LMWHs in animal models.[35] However andexanet alfa is not yet clinically available in the United States.

VITAMIN K ANTAGONISTS

A wide variety of vitamin K antagonists (VKAs) are available worldwide. The most widely prescribed and studied of these is warfarin. All VKAs work by inhibiting the vitamin K–dependent synthesis of factors II, VII, IX, and X in the liver.[36] Synthesis of the anticoagulant proteins C, S, and Z is also vitamin K dependent. Due to the short half-lives of these anticoagulant proteins in serum, initiation of VKA therapy without bridging may cause a transitory hypercoagulable state, which is undesirable in patients who are at intrinsically high risk of spontaneous thrombosis.[37]

Dosing of warfarin is inherently problematic due to dietary and drug-drug interactions (**Table 2**) and is best managed by a clinic experienced in the monitoring and dosing of VKAs. The international normalized ratio (INR) is the most validated study for monitoring VKA activity.[38]

Indications

VKAs are indicated in a wide variety of situations, from thromboembolism prophylaxis in patients with atrial fibrillation,[1] to secondary prevention of VTE,[39] to maintenance anticoagulation for patients with mechanical cardiac devices.[27]

Table 2
Medications that commonly interact with vitamin K antagonist dosing

Potentiate		
Antimicrobials	Cardiovascular	Other
Ciprofloxacin	Amiodarone	Acetaminophen
Erythromycin	Diltiazem	Aspirin
Fluconazole	Propanolol	Celecoxib
Cotrimoxazole	Simvastatin	Tramadol
Isoniazid		Phenytoin
Voriconazole		Ethanol
Metronidazole		Citalopram
		Sertraline
Inhibit		
Antimicrobials	Immune Modulators	Other
Ribavirin	Mesalamine	Carbemazepine
Rifampin	Azathioprine	Chlordiazepoxide
Nafcillin		

Kinetics

Warfarin is prepared as a racemic mixture of 2 enantiomers: R-warfarin and S-warfarin. The S-isoform is more potent. VKAs have excellent bioavailability after oral dosing. Time to peak concentration is observed to be approximately 90 minutes. The serum half-life is 36 hours to 42 hours.[40,41] The clinical effect is far more durable, however, due to potent and long-lasting inhibition of vitamin K epoxide reductase. Warfarin is highly bound to albumin in circulation. Metabolism of warfarin varies between isoforms. The R-isoform is more than 90% metabolized by CYP2C9 and CYP3A4. The S-isoform is approximately 60% metabolized by CYPs 1A2, 3A4, and 2C19. The remainder of clearance is by reductive metabolism to alcohols.

Interactions

Due to extensive metabolism by the cytochrome P-450 system, any genetic variations in the system or drugs that have an impact on activity of the system can have profound impacts on warfarin dosing or INR stability. See **Table 2** for a summary of drugs that commonly interact with warfarin.[42]

Other disease states, such as liver failure, tobacco use (due to induction of CYP1A2),[43] and end-stage renal disease (due to suppression of CYP2C9),[44] may also interfere with effective VKA dosing.

Adverse Effects

The most common adverse effects of VKAs are nontherapeutic INR and hemorrhage.[45] Patients who spend more time with a nontherapeutic INR are twice as likely to experience thrombotic and hemorrhagic complications[46] and the incidence of these complications is further affected by the target INR range, patient age, and adherence to a monitoring regime.[47] The most common hemorrhagic complications are gastrointestinal bleeding and hematuria.[48] The most feared complication, however, is spontaneous or traumatic intracerebral hemorrhage.

One of the most serious thrombotic complications of warfarin therapy is warfarin-induced skin necrosis, which occurs as a result of microvascular thrombosis concentrated in the capillaries and venules. This condition is highly morbid and often requires surgical intervention.[37]

Warfarin and other coumarins must not be administered to pregnant patients because more than one-third of pregnant patients experience unacceptable pregnancy outcomes, including bone agenesis and stillbirth.[49]

Reversal

Due to the high incidence of supratherapeutic INR and hemorrhage for patients on VKA therapy, an effective reversal strategy is necessary. A 4-tiered approach consisting of withholding the VKA, vitamin K, FFP, and PCCs can be envisioned.

For nonbleeding patients with supratherapeutic INR, either withholding the VKA alone or administering vitamin K as monotherapy may be sufficient to reverse VKA anticoagulation. For patients with INR 6.0 to 10.0, waiting alone sees an INR decrease below 4.0 in on average of 2.6 days.[50] If more rapid correction is desired, low-dose vitamin K, administered either orally or IV, corrects the INR to below 3.0 within 24 hours.[51] Oral to IV dosing conversion of vitamin K is 5:1, although IV dosing more frequently results in overcorrection. Subcutaneous dosing is not recommended due to unpredictable absorption.[52] Hepatic insufficiency may limit the efficacy of vitamin K–based reversal.

Because the coagulopathy of VKAs is due to deficiency of circulating, functional clotting factors, factor replacement is the cornerstone of reversal in hemorrhaging patients with supratherapeutic INR. FFP remains the most commonly used clotting factor replacement for patients on VKA with supratherapeutic INR.[45] FFP is inexpensive and widely available. It does carry an infectious risk, however, and the rate of transfusion-related acute lung injury (TRALI) is approximately 1 U in 5000 U transfused.[53] This may be an underestimate, however, due to poor reporting and underdiagnosis of TRALI. FFP therapy is further limited by the high volumes that may need to be transfused as well as delay in receiving these products from the blood bank due to the need for type-specific units and thawing of frozen units. FFP also has a short clinical half-life, necessitating redosing in some patients.

PCCs are a heterogeneous group of products that contain a mix of purified clotting factors. There are 3 large groups of products, all of which contain a mix of factors, in addition to varying amounts of heparin and proteins C and S. Three-factor PCCs (Profilnine [which does not contain heparin] [Grifols, Barcelona, Spain], and Bebulin VH [Baxter, Deerfield, Illinois] are available in the United States) contain proprietary concentrations of factors II, IX, and X. Four-factor PCCs (including Kcentra [CSL Behring, King of Prussia, Pennsylvania], which is available in the United States) contain factors II, VII, IX, and X. Activated 4-factor PCCs (FEIBA, Baxalta, Bannockburn, Illinois) contain activated factor VIIa, in addition to factors II, IX, and X. All preparations are dosed in a weight-based fashion based on factor IX. Because these products are heterogeneous, it is important to note the exact product being described in the literature as well as which exact products are available in an institution. Caution should be taken in administering heparin-containing PCCs to patients with proved HIT because some products contain small amounts of heparin.

PCCs are likely more effective in reversing the coagulopathy due to VKA therapy.[54] These products do not require ABO matching, are often immediately available, and can be quickly reconstituted and administered. Because they are purified and contain no living cells, the infective risk with PCCs is essentially nonexistent. In a prospective, randomized controlled trial of VKA reversal in hemorrhaging patients, 3-factor PCCs reliably reversed VKA anticoagulation within 30 minutes and the effect persisted for up to 24 hours.[55] The magnitude of correction was greater in the PCC group than the FFP group and hemostasis was better in the PCC group. The American College of Chest Physicians recommends PCC as the first-line therapy for hemorrhaging patients who have been taking VKAs.[54]

Recombinant activated factor VII (NovoSeven, Novo Nordisk, Bagsvaerd, Denmark) has been used to reverse VKA anticoagulation.[56] Insufficient prospective data, however, make it impossible to recommend its use for VKA reversal.

DIRECT THROMBIN INHIBITORS

The DTIs are a class of medications that do not require a cofactor to effect inhibition of thrombin. Four parenteral agents are approved in the United States: lepirudin, desirudin, bivalirudin, and argatroban. The oral agent dabigatran etexilate was approved by the Food and Drug Administration (FDA) in 2010.

Argatroban is a small, competitive thrombin antagonist. It is most commonly used for anticoagulation of patients with proved HIT and is also approved as an alternative to heparin during percutaneous interventions.[13]

Lepirudin and desirudin are hirudin derivatives. Hirudin is a 65 amino acid polypeptide isolated from the secretions of the medical leech *Hirudo medicinalis*. Lepirudin is only approved for the treatment of HIT-associated thrombosis.[10] Desirudin is only approved for VTE prophylaxis after hip replacement.[11]

Bivalirudin is a synthetic hirudin analog polypeptide that is 20 amino acids in length. Bivalirudin is approved for use as an alternative to heparin in patients undergoing percutaneous coronary interventions, specifically for those with HIT.[12]

Dabigatran etexilate is administered orally and is approved for stroke prevention in patients with nonvalvular atrial fibrillation and for both the acute treatment and secondary prevention of VTE.[57] The most common dosing regimens are 220 mg twice daily for those with normal renal function and 150 mg twice daily for patients with significant renal impairment.[14]

Monitoring

Several laboratory studies have been investigated for monitoring of DTI therapy and it seems that aPTT may be the most relevant. Ecarin clotting time may be more accurate than aPTT but this test is not widely available.[58] Routine laboratory monitoring, however, is not indicated.

Kinetics

All of the parenteral DTIs have excellent bioavailability after IV and subcutaneous administration. Half-life depends on the agent and route of administration.

- Argatroban: 30 to 50 minutes during continuous IV infusion; hepatic clearance[13]
- Bivalirudin: 25 minutes after IV administration, renal clearance[12]
- Desirudin: 2 hours after subcutaneous administration, 1 hour after IV administration; renal clearance[11]
- Lepirudin: 1 hour after IV administration; renal clearance[10]

Dabigatran has no bioavailability after oral administration so it is given as the prodrug dabigatran etexilate, which is converted to the active form by microsomal carboxylesterases in the liver.[57] Therefore, dabigatran's clinical effect depends intact hepatic upon metabolic function. Peak serum dabigatran concentrations are observed 2 hours after oral administration of dabigatran etexilate. Dabigatran is significantly redistributed to tissues after administration; 80% to 85% of dabigatran is excreted unchanged in the urine with the remainder metabolized by hepatic glucuronidation. The observed half-life is 8 hours to 13 hours depending on the population and dosing regimen. Decreased creatinine clearance significantly prolongs elimination. Dabigatran is effectively dialyzed.[57]

Reversal

No reversal agents exist for argatroban, bivalirudin, desirudin, or lepirudin.[59] This significantly limits the wider use of these agents.

Despite its widespread adoption after FDA approval, no proved reversal agent existed for dabigatran until the FDA-approved idarucizumab (Praxbind, Boehringer Ingelheim, Ingelheim am Rhein, Germany) in 2015. Idarucizumab is a humanized monoclonal antibody fragment that selectively binds dabigatran in a 1:1 stoichiometric ratio.[15] On-time is on the order of a few milliseconds whereas off-time is long enough to make binding essentially irreversible. Neither idarucizumab or the idarucizumab-dabigatran complex has intrinsic procoagulant or anticoagulant activity.[15]

Dose-response studies show that at even low doses, idarucizumab reverses the anticoagulant effect of dabigatran.[15] At doses less than 2 g, however, there is a rebound in the level of anticoagulation observed, likely due to redistribution of dabigatran from the nonvascular to the vascular compartment. Therefore, doses of at least 2 g are recommended. Idarucizumab comes reconstituted in solution in a package of two 2.5-g vials. It is typically administered as a total dose of 5 g given in split doses no more than 15 minutes apart.

Idarucizmab and the idarucizumab-dabigatran complex are both renally cleared. Given that idarucizumab is orders of magnitude more massive than dabigatran, it is not surprising that binding to dabigatran does not affect clearance of the compound.[15] Idarucizumab is virtually undetectable in the serum 4 hours after administration.

The largest clinical study of idarucizumab reversal of dabigatran is the REVERSE-AD trial,[60] of which results for the first 90 patients were published in 2015. In this prospective cohort trial, patients on dabigatran who either had life-threatening hemorrhage (ICH, gastrointestinal bleeding, and so forth) or presented for emergent or urgent surgery, which could not be delayed (trauma, acute cholecystectomy, and so forth), received a 5-g dose of idarucizumab. The investigators showed impressive laboratory reversal of coagulation abnormalities in both groups. A majority of patients in the surgical group had normal intraoperative hemostasis. Five significant thrombotic events were reported in this trial. All thromboses occurred more than 48 hours after idarucizumab administration, however, and in the absence of any therapeutic or prophylactic anticoagulation, making it unlikely that they were directly related to idarucizumab administration.[60]

Studies have shown that some patients make antibodies in response to idarucizumab administration. To date, however, no neutralizing antibodies have been reported.[60] The most common reported side effects are headache, nasopharyngitis, back pain, and skin irritation.

DIRECT FACTOR XA INHIBITORS

Three new agents in the class — rivaroxaban (Xarelto, Bayer, Leverkusen, Germany), apixaban (Eliquis, Bristol-Myers Squibb, New York, New York), and edoxaban (Savaysa, Daiichi Sankyo, Tokyo, Japan) — are available in the United States and a fourth, betrixaban (Portola Pharmaceuticals, South San Francisco, California) is still in development. All of these agents specifically and directly inhibit function of activated factor X by noncovalent bonding.[16–18]

Every agent in this class is given orally. The most common dosing regimens are

- Rivaroxaban: 20 mg daily for VTE and stroke prophylaxis, 15 mg twice daily for treatment of VTE[16]
- Apixaban: 2.5 mg to 5 mg twice daily for VTE and stroke prophylaxis, 10 mg twice daily for treatment of VTE[17]
- Edoxaban: 30 mg to 60 mg daily depending on indication[18]

Indications

Rivaroxaban and apixaban are both FDA approved for stroke prevention in nonvalvular atrial fibrillation, treatment and secondary prevention of VTE, and VTE prophylaxis after major orthopedic surgery.[16,17] Edoxaban is FDA approved only in patients with renal impairment for stroke prevention in nonvalvular atrial fibrillation and for acute treatment of VTE.[18]

Kinetics

All agents in this class have excellent bioavailability after oral administration. They also have large volumes of distribution (50–100 L, depending on the agent and body habitus of the patient) due to high fractions of protein binding, mainly to albumin. Only the free, unbound drug is pharmacologically active.

- Time to peak effect for rivaroxaban is observed to be 2 hours to 4 hours and elimination half-time is 5 hours to 11 hours. The compound is primarily metabolized by CYP3A4, although it does not seem to induce or inhibit hepatic enzymes and is then cleared primarily by the kidneys. Elimination is prolonged in patients with renal dysfunction. Rivaroxaban is not dialyzable.[61]
- Apixaban's peak effect is observed 3 hours to 4 hours after administration. This compound is also metabolized by CPY3A4, but primary clearance is by biliary and enteric excretion. Apixaban is poorly dialyzable and its elimination is prolonged in patients with hepatic dysfunction.[62]
- Edoxaban has a time of to peak effect of 1 hour to 2 hours after oral administration and an elimination half-time of 10 hours to 14 hours. There is some spontaneous hydrolysis of edoxaban in the serum and 1 metabolite, M-4, is active. Edoxaban is primarily excreted unchanged in the biliary and renal systems. Significant renal dysfunction does not prolong elimination. Edoxaban is not dialyzable.[18]

Monitoring

Of the commonly available laboratory tests, it seems that prothrombin time or INR may be the most sensitive to the effect of oral Xa inhibitors. The diluted Russell viper venom ratio may be the preferred test for monitoring because there is a predictable dose-response effect. This test is not widely available, however. Anti-Xa activity assays do not seem to be effective for monitoring.[63]

Reversal

At this time there are no FDA-approved agents for the reversal of direct Xa inhibitors. Several agents, however, some of which are commercially available, have been investigated as antidotes for compounds in this class.

Prothrombin Complex Concentrates

In theory, large amounts of clotting factor, such as those administered with higher doses of PCC, may be able to overcome the upstream inhibition imposed by direct Xa inhibitors. Human volunteer studies show that it may be possible to correct some of the coagulation abnormalities associated with direct Xa inhibition.[64] Animal models also suggest that it is possible to slow hematoma growth with PCC administration.[65,66] No prospective human clinical trials have been published, however, on this subject and PCC reversal of oral Xa inhibitors remains off-label.

Andexanet Alfa

Andexanet alfa is an investigational compound being developed by Portola Pharmaceuticals for the reversal of anticoagulation due to Xa inhibition. In theory, it should be effective with heparins and LMWHs as well as oral direct Xa inhibitors. This agent is a truncated Xa analog that sequesters anticoagulants and prevents them from binding to factor Xa. Binding is noncovalent and reversible. Safety studies suggest that neither andexanet-alfa nor the andexanet alfa-apixaban/rivaroxaban complex has intrinsic procoagulant or anticoagulant activity.[35,67]

Dose-response studies suggest that the dose of andexanet depends on the agent being reversed[67]:

- Apixaban: 400-mg IV bolus plus 4 mg/min IV continuous infusion
- Rivaroxaban: 800-mg IV bolus plus 8 mg/min IV continuous infusion
- Dose-response data for edoxaban have not yet been published.

Kinetics

Peak effect with andexanet is observed almost immediately after bolus dosing. In dose-response studies, it was observed that the reversal effect was transient after bolus dosing as clotting studies returned to anticoagulated baseline within 1 hour to 2 hours if the patients did not receive a continuous infusion.[67] As such, a continuous infusion is likely mandatory in the clinical setting. In these studies, the subjects in the bolus-plus-infusion groups saw the reversal effect maintained as long as the infusion was continued. The reversal effect ceased soon after discontinuing the infusion. No data have been published in a peer-reviewed journal regarding the clearance of andexanet alfa.

In the ANNEXA-A and ANNEXA-R trials, 1 patient had hives after andexanet alfa infusion. No thrombotic events or anti-X/Xa antibodies were reported; 17 of 101 patients developed non-neutralizing antibodies against andexanet alfa, but no neutralizing antibodies were reported.[67]

Availability

Phase III trials are currently ongoing and FDA approval of andexanet alfa is pending the results of these studies. This medication is currently unavailable in the United States except for investigational purposes.

Cirapirantag

Cirapirantag (formerly known as PER977 or apirazine) (Perosphere, Danbury, Connecticut) is an investigational compound that has been granted fast-track status by the FDA. This substance nonspecifically, noncovalently binds to heparin, LMWH, direct Xa inhibitors, and DTIs and has the ability to sequester all of these compounds, thereby neutralizing their anticoagulant effects. In animal models, thrombography showed that Cirapirantag reversed the anticoagulant effect of all of these medications. In a human volunteer study of 80 healthy patients published as correspondence in *The New England Journal of Medicine*, it was shown that a single dose of cirapirantag readily reversed the anticoagulant effect of edoxaban to a nonanticoagulated baseline and that there was greater fibrin polymerization in those that received the study drug.[68] No larger studies or dose-response studies have yet been published. Cirapirantag is not yet available in the United States.

APPLICATIONS FOR THE ANESTHESIOLOGIST

Patients needing reversal of anticoagulation should be thought of as belonging to 2 distinct groups: those with life-threatening hemorrhage and those on maintenance anticoagulation who present for surgery. These patients are intrinsically different from those with consumptive coagulopathy because specific agents, and not empiric or goal-directed transfusion, are needed to correct the coagulopathy. Additionally, there is a subset of patients — those with mechanical cardiac devices, such as mechanical valves, VADs, or ECMO support — on maintenance anticoagulation for whom it may not safe to reverse the anticoagulant effect.

For patients who are not bleeding but whose procedure cannot be delayed, a rational approach is recommended. Time alone may be adequate to ensure sufficient reversal because several anticoagulants — unfractionated heparin, parenteral DTIs — should be spontaneously reversed within 2 hours to 4 hours. Other agents with more durable clinical effects may be too long-lasting for waiting to be practical, such as in patients on warfarin who present for fixation of traumatic femur fracture. In these cases, it is reasonable to administer a reversal agent. The choice of agent should be specific to the compound being reversed, and laboratory guidance may be helpful in guiding therapy. Patients coming from home for elective surgeries, however, for whom it safe to stop anticoagulation, should be asked to stop their medication and allow the anticoagulant effect to resolve before proceeding to the operating room. Laboratory guidance may be helpful.

The bigger challenge comes in treating patients who are already hemorrhaging as a combination of antidote and clotting factor replacement may be necessary to both reverse the anticoagulant and treat the consumptive coagulopathy. Again, reversal agents — due to their cost and adverse effects — should only be given if it is known or thought highly likely that a patient has been taking the offending agent. At this time, high doses of 4-factor PCCs are the only available product to reverse direct Xa inhibitors and are reasonable to administer in this situation, despite the lack of prospective data. No potent reversal agents are available for LMWH or parenteral DTIs.

Possibly the most complex situation arises when a patient with a durable mechanical cardiac device, such as a mechanical heart valve or VAD, presents for neurologic surgery, specifically intracranial and spinal procedures where the consequences of even small-volume bleeding may be catastrophic. Case reports suggest that is likely safe to suspend anticoagulation for a brief period. These patients are best managed as inpatients before surgery. Their warfarin should be bridged to heparin and they should be maintained on heparin until warfarin's clinical effect is resolved. This may take 3 days to 7 days. Heparin may be stopped shortly (0–2 hours) before going to the operating room and resumed as soon as possible after the procedure. Close coordination with neurosurgeons, cardiologists, and even hematologists as well as patients is necessary to ensure the best possible outcomes for these patients. If the risks of stopping anticoagulation are too high, it may not be possible for a patient to have surgery.

REFERENCES

1. You JJ, Singer DE, Howard PA, et al. Antithrombotic therapy for atrial fibrillation: Antithrombotic therapy and prevention of thrombosis, 9th ed: American college of chest physicians evidence-based clinical practice guidelines. Chest 2012; 141(2 Suppl):e531S–75S.
2. Kearon C, Akl EA, Comerota AJ, et al. Antithrombotic therapy for VTE disease: Antithrombotic therapy and prevention of thrombosis, 9th ed: American college of chest physicians evidence-based clinical practice guidelines. Chest 2012; 141(2 Suppl):e419S–94S.
3. Alonso-Coello P, Bellmunt S, McGorrian C, et al. Antithrombotic therapy in peripheral artery disease: antithrombotic therapy and prevention of thrombosis, 9th ed: American college of chest physicians evidence-based clinical practice guidelines. Chest 2012;141(2 Suppl):e669S–90S.
4. Palareti G, Leali N, Coccheri S, et al. Bleeding complications of oral anticoagulant treatment: An inception-cohort, prospective collaborative study (ISCOAT). italian study on complications of oral anticoagulant therapy. Lancet 1996;348(9025):423–8.
5. Young EY, Ahmadinia K, Bajwa N, et al. Does chronic warfarin cause increased blood loss and transfusion during lumbar spinal surgery? Spine J 2013;13(10): 1253–8.
6. Heparin sodium [package insert]. Lake Forest, IL: Hospira, Inc; 2013.
7. Enoxaparin sodium (lovenox (r)) [package insert]. Bridgewater, NJ: Sanofi-aventis US, LLC; 2013.
8. Fondaparinux (arixtra (r)) [package insert]. Concord, Ontario, Canada: Aspri Pharma Canada; 2015.

9. Warfarin (coumadin (r)) [package insert]. Princeton, NJ: Bristol-Myers Squibb; 2015.
10. Lepirudin [package insert]. Marburg, Germany: ZLB Behring GmbH; 2004.
11. Desirudin [package insert]. Northbrook, IL: Marathon Pharmaceuticals; 2013.
12. Bivalirudin [package insert]. Marlborough, MA: Sunovion Pharmaceuticals; 2016.
13. Argatroban [package insert]. GlaxoSmithKline, Research Triangle Park; 2016.
14. Dabigatran etexilate (pradaxa (r)) [package insert]. Ingelheim Am Rhein, Germany: Boehringer Ingelheim Pharmaceuticals; 2015.
15. Glund S, Moschetti V, Norris S, et al. A randomised study in healthy volunteers to investigate the safety, tolerability and pharmacokinetics of idarucizumab, a specific antidote to dabigatran. Thromb Haemost 2015;113(5):943–51.
16. Rivaroxaban [package insert]. Leverkusen, Germany: Bayer Pharma AG; 2016.
17. Apixaban [package insert]. New York, NY: Bristol-Meyers Squibb; 2016.
18. Edoxaban [package insert]. Tokyo, Japan: Daiichi Sankyo; 2015.
19. Rosenberg RD, Lam L. Correlation between structure and function of heparin. Proc Natl Acad Sci U S A 1979;76(3):1218–22.
20. Abildgaard U. Highly purified antithrombin 3 with heparin cofactor activity prepared by disc electrophoresis. Scand J Clin Lab Invest 1968;21(1):89–91.
21. Francis JL, Palmer GJ 3rd, Moroose R, et al. Comparison of bovine and porcine heparin in heparin antibody formation after cardiac surgery. Ann Thorac Surg 2003;75(1):17–22.
22. Basu D, Gallus A, Hirsh J, et al. A prospective study of the value of monitoring heparin treatment with the activated partial thromboplastin time. N Engl J Med 1972;287(7):324–7.
23. Choay J, Lormeau JC, Petitou M, et al. Anti-xa active heparin oligosaccharides. Thromb Res 1980;18(3–4):573–8.
24. Frydman AM, Bara L, Le Roux Y, et al. The antithrombotic activity and pharmacokinetics of enoxaparine, a low molecular weight heparin, in humans given single subcutaneous doses of 20 to 80 mg. J Clin Pharmacol 1988;28(7):609–18.
25. Warkentin TE, Levine MN, Hirsh J, et al. Heparin-induced thrombocytopenia in patients treated with low-molecular-weight heparin or unfractionated heparin. N Engl J Med 1995;332(20):1330–5.
26. Bounameaux H, Perneger T. Fondaparinux: A new synthetic pentasaccharide for thrombosis prevention. Lancet 2002;359(9319):1710–1.
27. Whitlock RP, Sun JC, Fremes SE, et al. American College of Chest Physicians. Antithrombotic and thrombolytic therapy for valvular disease: Antithrombotic therapy and prevention of thrombosis, 9th ed: American college of chest physicians evidence-based clinical practice guidelines. Chest 2012;141(2 Suppl): e576S–600S.
28. Bjornsson TD, Wolfram KM, Kitchell BB. Heparin kinetics determined by three assay methods. Clin Pharmacol Ther 1982;31(1):104–13.
29. Olsson P, Lagergren H, Ek S. The elimination from plasma of intravenous heparin. an experimental study on dogs and humans. Acta Med Scand 1963;173:619–30.
30. Donat H, Ozcan A. Comparison of the effectiveness of two programmes on older adults at risk of falling: Unsupervised home exercise and supervised group exercise. Clin Rehabil 2007;21(3):273–83.
31. Protamine sulfate [package insert]. Schaumberg, IL: Fresenius Kabi USA, LLC; 2008.
32. Caplan SN, Berkman EM. Letter: Protamine sulfate and fish allergy. N Engl J Med 1976;295(3):172.

33. Massonnet-Castel S, Pelissier E, Bara L, et al. Partial reversal of low molecular weight heparin (PK 10169) anti-xa activity by protamine sulfate: In vitro and in vivo study during cardiac surgery with extracorporeal circulation. Haemostasis 1986;16(2):139–46.
34. Garcia DA, Baglin TP, Weitz JI, et al. American College of Chest Physicians. Parenteral anticoagulants: Antithrombotic therapy and prevention of thrombosis, 9th ed: American college of chest physicians evidence-based clinical practice guidelines. Chest 2012;141(2 Suppl):e24S–43S.
35. Lu G, DeGuzman FR, Hollenbach SJ, et al. A specific antidote for reversal of anticoagulation by direct and indirect inhibitors of coagulation factor xa. Nat Med 2013;19(4):446–51.
36. Whitlon DS, Sadowski JA, Suttie JW. Mechanism of coumarin action: Significance of vitamin K epoxide reductase inhibition. Biochemistry 1978;17(8):1371–7.
37. Weinberg AC, Lieskovsky G, McGehee WG, et al. Warfarin necrosis of the skin and subcutaneous tissue of the male external genitalia. J Urol 1983;130(2):352–4.
38. Friedman PA, Rosenberg RD, Hauschka PV, et al. A spectrum of partially carboxylated prothrombins in the plasmas of coumarin-treated patients. Biochim Biophys Acta 1977;494(1):271–6.
39. Gould MK, Garcia DA, Wren SM, et al. Prevention of VTE in nonorthopedic surgical patients: Antithrombotic therapy and prevention of thrombosis, 9th ed: American college of chest physicians evidence-based clinical practice guidelines. Chest 2012;141(2 Suppl):e227S–77S.
40. Breckenridge A. Oral anticoagulant drugs: Pharmacokinetic aspects. Semin Hematol 1978;15(1):19–26.
41. Kelly JG, O'Malley K. Clinical pharmacokinetics of oral anticoagulants. Clin Pharmacokinet 1979;4(1):1–15.
42. Holbrook AM, Pereira JA, Labiris R, et al. Systematic overview of warfarin and its drug and food interactions. Arch Intern Med 2005;165(10):1095–106.
43. Gunes A, Dahl ML. Variation in CYP1A2 activity and its clinical implications: Influence of environmental factors and genetic polymorphisms. Pharmacogenomics 2008;9(5):625–37.
44. Dreisbach AW, Japa S, Gebrekal AB, et al. Cytochrome P4502C9 activity in end-stage renal disease. Clin Pharmacol Ther 2003;73(5):475–7.
45. Ageno W, Garcia D, Aguilar MI, et al. Prevention and treatment of bleeding complications in patients receiving vitamin K antagonists, part 2: Treatment. Am J Hematol 2009;84(9):584–8.
46. White HD, Gruber M, Feyzi J, et al. Comparison of outcomes among patients randomized to warfarin therapy according to anticoagulant control: Results from SPORTIF III and V. Arch Intern Med 2007;167(3):239–45.
47. van der Meer FJ, Rosendaal FR, Vandenbroucke JP, et al. Bleeding complications in oral anticoagulant therapy. an analysis of risk factors. Arch Intern Med 1993;153(13):1557–62.
48. Bjorck F, Renlund H, Lip GY, et al. Outcomes in a warfarin-treated population with atrial fibrillation. JAMA Cardiol 2016;1(2):172–80.
49. Hall JG, Pauli RM, Wilson KM. Maternal and fetal sequelae of anticoagulation during pregnancy. Am J Med 1980;68(1):122–40.
50. Patel RJ, Witt DM, Saseen JJ, et al. Randomized, placebo-controlled trial of oral phytonadione for excessive anticoagulation. Pharmacotherapy 2000;20(10):1159–66.

51. Lubetsky A, Yonath H, Olchovsky D, et al. Comparison of oral vs intravenous phytonadione (vitamin K1) in patients with excessive anticoagulation: A prospective randomized controlled study. Arch Intern Med 2003;163(20):2469–73.
52. Crowther MA, Douketis JD, Schnurr T, et al. Oral vitamin K lowers the international normalized ratio more rapidly than subcutaneous vitamin K in the treatment of warfarin-associated coagulopathy. A randomized, controlled trial. Ann Intern Med 2002;137(4):251–4.
53. Popovsky MA. Transfusion-related acute lung injury: Incidence, pathogenesis and the role of multicomponent apheresis in its prevention. Transfus Med Hemother 2008;35(2):76–9.
54. Ageno W, Gallus AS, Wittkowsky A, et al. Oral anticoagulant therapy: Antithrombotic therapy and prevention of thrombosis, 9th ed: American college of chest physicians evidence-based clinical practice guidelines. Chest 2012;141(2 Suppl): e44S–88S.
55. Boulis NM, Bobek MP, Schmaier A, et al. Use of factor IX complex in warfarin-related intracranial hemorrhage. Neurosurgery 1999;45(5):1113–8 [discussion: 1118–9].
56. Ilyas C, Beyer GM, Dutton RP, et al. Recombinant factor VIIa for warfarin-associated intracranial bleeding. J Clin Anesth 2008;20(4):276–9.
57. Stangier J. Clinical pharmacokinetics and pharmacodynamics of the oral direct thrombin inhibitor dabigatran etexilate. Clin Pharmacokinet 2008;47(5):285–95.
58. van Ryn J, Stangier J, Haertter S, et al. Dabigatran etexilate–a novel, reversible, oral direct thrombin inhibitor: Interpretation of coagulation assays and reversal of anticoagulant activity. Thromb Haemost 2010;103(6):1116–27.
59. Greinacher A, Thiele T, Selleng K. Reversal of anticoagulants: An overview of current developments. Thromb Haemost 2015;113(5):931–42.
60. Pollack CV Jr, Reilly PA, Eikelboom J, et al. Idarucizumab for dabigatran reversal. N Engl J Med 2015;373(6):511–20.
61. Kubitza D, Becka M, Voith B, et al. Safety, pharmacodynamics, and pharmacokinetics of single doses of BAY 59-7939, an oral, direct factor xa inhibitor. Clin Pharmacol Ther 2005;78(4):412–21.
62. Frost C, Nepal S, Wang J, et al. Safety, pharmacokinetics and pharmacodynamics of multiple oral doses of apixaban, a factor xa inhibitor, in healthy subjects. Br J Clin Pharmacol 2013;76(5):776–86.
63. Samama MM, Martinoli JL, LeFlem L, et al. Assessment of laboratory assays to measure rivaroxaban–an oral, direct factor xa inhibitor. Thromb Haemost 2010; 103(4):815–25.
64. Barco S, Whitney Cheung Y, Coppens M, et al. In vivo reversal of the anticoagulant effect of rivaroxaban with four-factor prothrombin complex concentrate. Br J Haematol 2016;172(2):255–61.
65. Herzog E, Kaspereit F, Krege W, et al. Correlation of coagulation markers and 4F-PCC-mediated reversal of rivaroxaban in a rabbit model of acute bleeding. Thromb Res 2015;135(3):554–60.
66. Perzborn E, Gruber A, Tinel H, et al. Reversal of rivaroxaban anticoagulation by haemostatic agents in rats and primates. Thromb Haemost 2013;110(1):162–72.
67. Siegal DM, Curnutte JT, Connolly SJ, et al. Andexanet alfa for the reversal of factor xa inhibitor activity. N Engl J Med 2015;373(25):2413–24.
68. Ansell JE, Bakhru SH, Laulicht BE, et al. Use of PER977 to reverse the anticoagulant effect of edoxaban. N Engl J Med 2014;371(22):2141–2.

Uterotonic Medications

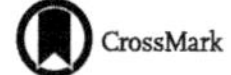

Oxytocin, Methylergonovine, Carboprost, Misoprostol

Cristianna Vallera, MD*, Lynn O. Choi, MD,
Catherine M. Cha, MD, Richard W. Hong, MD

KEYWORDS

- Oxytocin • Methylergonovine • Carboprost • Misoprostol • Uterine atony
- Uterotonic agent • Postpartum hemorrhage

KEY POINTS

- Uterotonic agents are widely used in the prevention and treatment of postpartum hemorrhage, and although oxytocin remains the first-line agent, a standardized guideline for optimal dose and rate of administration has not been clearly defined.
- Methylergonovine is a highly effective second-line agent; however, it is associated with severe vasoconstriction and is contraindicated for hypertensive patients.
- Carboprost is useful for escalation of treatment when oxytocin and uterine massage have been insufficient to restore uterine tone, especially when methylergonovine is contraindicated, but it can cause severe bronchospasm and is thus contraindicated in patients with asthma.
- Misoprostol is characterized by low cost, stability in storage, broad availability, minimal side effects, ease of administration, and multiple medical uses; however, recent studies have called into question its effectiveness as an adjunct uterotonic agent, limiting its role to scenarios in which other, injectable uterotonics are not readily available or easily administered.

OXYTOCIN

Introduction

Oxytocin, the first-line agent in the prevention and treatment of postpartum hemorrhage, is a polypeptide structure that is produced in the paraventricular nucleus of the hypothalamus and released by the posterior pituitary gland. It was first discovered by Sir Henry Dale in 1909 when he discovered that a hormone from the pituitary gland

Disclosure Statement: The authors have nothing to disclose.
Department of Anesthesiology and Perioperative Medicine, David Geffen School of Medicine at UCLA, 757 Westwood Plaza, Suite 3325, Los Angeles, CA 90095-7403, USA
* Corresponding author.
E-mail address: cvallera@mednet.ucla.edu

Anesthesiology Clin 35 (2017) 207–219
http://dx.doi.org/10.1016/j.anclin.2017.01.007

caused uterine contractions in a pregnant cat.[1] It was the first polypeptide hormone synthesized in 1953 by the American biochemist, Vincent Du Vigneaud.[2] Oxytocin remains the first-line agent in the management and prevention of uterine atony after vaginal and operative delivery. The clinical roles of oxytocin in the obstetric population include induction and augmentation of labor, and prevention and treatment of postpartum uterine atony.

Structure/Activity

Oxytocin is a short polypeptide consisting of 9 peptides (nonapeptide). Its chemical structure is $C_{46}H_{66}N_{12}O_{12}S_2$, which is structurally similar to vasopressin, and both are secreted by the posterior pituitary gland. A disulfide bridge connects 2 cystines in the primary sequence (Cys1 and Cys 6), forming a ring.[3]

Oxytocin exerts a stimulatory effect on myometrial contractility by increasing the intracellular concentration of calcium. This process is achieved by the release of calcium in the sarcoplasmic reticulum and by enhanced entry of extracellular calcium. Oxytocin binds to a G-protein on the surface of the uterine myocyte, resulting in the generation of diacylglycerol (DAG) and inositol triphosphate (IP3) via phospholipase C on phosphatidyl-inositol bisphosphate.[4] DAG stimulates prostaglandin synthesis, which also contributes to uterine contractions. IP3 stimulates the release of calcium from the sarcoplasmic reticulum and increases the concentration of cytoplasmic calcium.[5] For sufficient activation of myometrial contraction, this increase in intracellular calcium from the sarcoplasmic reticulum alone is not sufficient and entry of extracellular calcium is required. This process is mediated by the oxytocin–G-protein complex, which causes a conformational change in voltage-gated calcium channels allowing the influx of extracellular calcium. Calcium then binds to calmodulin and activates myosin light-chain kinase, which is the fundamental contraction mechanism of uterine smooth muscle.[6]

The rate-limiting step for the action of oxytocin is the concentration of oxytocin receptors on the myometrium. Of note, the oxytocin receptor is absent in a nonpregnant uterus. Once a woman becomes pregnant, oxytocin receptors appear in myometrial cells at approximately 13 weeks' gestation and increase in concentration until term. The distribution of oxytocin receptors in the uterus is not uniform throughout. There is a higher concentration of receptors in the fundus of the uterus, and the concentration decreases closer to the lower uterine segment and cervix.[5] This uneven receptor distribution may explain the less prominent uterine contraction seen in the lower third of the uterus after administration of oxytocin.

Pharmacokinetics

Oxytocin is absorbed via intravenous, intramuscular, buccal, or nasal mucosal routes, but it is most commonly administered intravenously to allow for precise dosing and rapid discontinuation if adverse reactions occur. Intravenous injection has an immediate onset of action compared with intramuscular injection, which takes approximately 3 to 7 minutes.[7] The recommended dose for intramuscular injection during cesarean delivery is 10 units after delivery of the placenta. Once absorbed, oxytocin redistributes to the extracellular space and does not bind to plasma proteins. The half-life of oxytocin is 10 to 12 minutes. There is a linear increase in plasma concentration of oxytocin after a continuous infusion. It takes approximately 20 to 30 minutes to reach a steady-state in plasma,[8] and a maximum concentration is reached in approximately 40 minutes.[9]

Although the mechanism of oxytocin degradation is not clearly elucidated, there are 2 proposed pathways that contribute to oxytocin metabolism, which involve cysteine aminopeptidase and postproline endopeptidase. Aminopeptidase splits the ring structure of oxytocin by cleaving tyrosine and destroys the conformational active state. Postproline endopeptidase cleaves oxytocin between proline and leucine, splitting the molecule into 2 inactive moieties. There are other minor enzymes involved in inactivating oxytocin, which include carboxypeptidase and leucine aminopeptidase.[10]

Clinical Role

Uterine atony is the most common cause of severe postpartum hemorrhage. Consequently, the use of uterotonic agents is crucial to reducing the risk of postpartum hemorrhage and improving maternal safety. Oxytocin is the drug of choice for prevention and treatment of uterine atony after vaginal and operative deliveries. It is also widely used to induce and augment the labor process.

Routes and Dosages

The dosage and method of administration of oxytocin for prevention and treatment of uterine atony vary considerably and remain controversial. The recommended routes for administration are intravenous or intramuscular. A Cochrane review comparing the administration of prophylactic oxytocin for postpartum hemorrhage found no difference in efficacy or side effects when comparing intravenous and intramuscular administration.[7] Potentially detrimental cardiovascular side effects are related to the dose and rate of administration. Rapid intravenous bolus injections of up to 3 to 5 units have resulted in cardiovascular collapse and even death.[11] In a study by Carvalho and colleagues,[12] the ED_{90} for nonlaboring patients undergoing elective cesarean delivery was found to be 0.35 units. Balki and colleagues[13] studied laboring women who required cesarean delivery for labor arrest that had been induced or augmented with oxytocin for approximately 10 hours and found that the ED_{90} was 2.99 units. Balki and his colleagues[13] demonstrated that the requirement for oxytocin in patients who were already exposed to oxytocin had about 9 times the requirement of nonlaboring patients.

There are several concepts that contribute to the different dosage requirements in laboring versus nonlaboring patients. Oxytocin receptor expression and density in the myometrium increases progressively throughout pregnancy and reaches a peak at term.[14] The change in receptor density explains why patients with term, elective cesarean deliveries are more sensitive to low dosages of oxytocin.[12]

Labor and oxytocin exposure further changes oxytocin receptor distribution. Phaneuf and colleagues[15] found that oxytocin receptor density was significantly lower in patients who had been induced with oxytocin compared with those who had spontaneous onset of labor. Repeated exposure of the myometrial cells to oxytocin leads to a significant loss in the capacity to respond to additional oxytocin, which is likely due to oxytocin receptor desensitization. Repeated doses of oxytocin may become increasingly ineffective and second-line uterotonics (ergometrine, prostaglandins $F2\alpha$ and E1) should be considered earlier for laboring patients, especially in those who have received oxytocin.

The recommended dose, timing, and rate of administration for oxytocin during cesarean delivery remain ambiguous. A randomized, double-blind study by Kovecheva and colleagues[16] used a "Rule of Threes" algorithm to minimize the dose-related and rate-related side effects of oxytocin by applying a standardized method of administering oxytocin during elective cesarean deliveries. The algorithm starts with an initial 3 units of oxytocin given over 5 seconds after delivery of the fetus, and uterine tone is assessed every 3 minutes thereafter. An additional 3 units of oxytocin is given if inadequate tone is observed after each 3-minute interval. If a third bolus of oxytocin is given for inadequate tone and uterine atony continues, then a second-line uterotonic agent is recommended. The "Rule of Threes" algorithm minimizes the total dose of oxytocin administered and may represent an optimal regimen for elective cesarean deliveries.

Side Effects and Contraindications

Oxytocin used for prophylaxis or treatment of postpartum hemorrhage during cesarean delivery may result in several side effects. The adverse effects include hemodynamic instability (hypotension, tachycardia, myocardial ischemia, and arrhythmias), nausea, vomiting, headache, and flushing. The most common side effects are hypotension and tachycardia and are related to the dose and rate of administration. Hypotension is predominately caused by transient relaxation of vascular smooth muscle cells via calcium-dependent stimulation of the nitric oxide pathway, which leads to peripheral vasodilation, hypotension, and a compensatory increase in heart rate, stroke volume, and cardiac output.[17] These cardiovascular effects may be well tolerated in a healthy patient but caution must be taken when administering to patients with abnormal ventricular function, valvular stenosis, or hypovolemia.[4] Due to its structural similarity to vasopressin, oxytocin administered in high dosages may lead to water intoxication, hyponatremia, seizures, and coma.[18]

Summary

Oxytocin remains the first-line agent for prevention and treatment of postpartum hemorrhage after vaginal and cesarean delivery. Adverse side effects leading to cardiovascular instability are dose and rate related. Currently, there are no standardized administration guidelines for the administration of oxytocin, but a "Rule of Threes" algorithm may be a safe method for oxytocin use during elective cesarean deliveries. Although oxytocin has been used safely and effectively by obstetricians and anesthesiologists for many years, the benefits of oxytocin must be weighed against potentially serious side effects.

METHYLERGONOVINE

Introduction

Methylergonovine has a long history of use for the treatment of postpartum hemorrhage due to uterine atony. It is a semisynthetic amide ergot derivative, which produces sustained contraction of the uterus without causing significant systemic vasoconstriction in most cases.[19] The American College of Obstetricians and Gynecologists recommends methylergonovine as a second-line uterotonic for refractory uterine atony.[20] However, in 2012, the Food and Drug Administration (FDA) raised potential safety concerns about methylergonovine-induced vasoconstriction causing myocardial ischemia and infarction, which led to a revision of the methylergonovine label.[21]

Structure/Activity

Ergot alkaloids were first isolated from ergot fungi and are derivatives of the tetracyclic compound 6-methylergoline.[19] Methylergonovine maleate (9,10-didehydro-N-[(S)-(1-hydroxymethyl) propyl]-6-methylergoline-8beta-carboxamide maleate salt) is a semisynthetic ergot alkaloid that is produced by a reaction of (+)-lysergic acid with L-(+)-aminobutanol.[22] Methylergonovine has low water solubility and is prepared as a water-soluble maleate salt.[23] Exposure to water or light leads to the formation of 6-hydroxy derivatives, which will be expedited in an acidic environment. It is easily oxidized, and the oxidation produces a color change. Methylergonovine should be administered only if it is clear and colorless. When stored, methylergonovine should be refrigerated. Stability is compromised when exposed to higher temperatures, light, or humidity.[19,22]

Methylergonovine is a serotonergic receptor agonist in the smooth muscle. It is also a weak antagonist of dopaminergic receptors and partial agonist of α-adrenergic receptors.[22] Methylergonovine causes uterine contractions and relaxation at low doses, but causes sustained contractions and increased basal tone at high doses.[24] The mechanism of action for uterine contraction is not well defined. Uterine contraction is likely produced by methylergonovine agonist effects on the 5-HT2 receptor found in uterine smooth muscle.[22] Alternatively, methylergonovine could cause uterine contraction through direct stimulation of the α-adrenergic receptors in the uterus, which has been postulated to lead to calcium mobilization.[25]

Pharmacokinetics

The onset of action of intravenous methylergonovine is nearly immediate. After intramuscular injection, the onset is 2 to 5 minutes, and after oral administration the onset is 5 to 10 minutes. If administered intravenously, methylergonovine is distributed from plasma to peripheral tissue in 2 to 3 minutes. Peak plasma concentration following intramuscular injection occurs in approximately 0.4 hour, and occurs approximately 1 hour after oral administration. Plasma levels have a biphasic decline with intramuscular absorption.[21] The half-life of methylergonovine after intravenous administration is 2.3 hours and after oral administration is 2.7 hours. The bioavailability is significantly more variable with oral administration when compared with intravenous or intramuscular administration.[22] Intramuscular injection had a greater bioavailability than oral administration, likely due to first-pass metabolism by the liver. Ergot alkaloids are mainly eliminated by hepatic metabolism.[21]

Clinical Role

Methylergonovine is used for the treatment postpartum hemorrhage due to uterine atony or subinvolution. At high doses, it creates sustained contractions in the uterus.[23,24] The American College of Obstetricians and Gynecologists (ACOG) recommends methylergonovine as a second-line uterotonic.[20] When compared with carboprost, methylergonovine has been associated with reduced risk of hemorrhage-related morbidity in women with uterine atony refractory to oxytocin.[26] Recently, methylergonovine has also been used to treat migraines and cluster headaches and to produce diagnostic coronary vasospasm in patients with variant angina.[24,27]

Route and Dosage

ACOG recommends methylergonovine at a dosage of 0.2 mg administered intramuscularly at a frequency of 2 to 4 hours as needed. ACOG also discusses some practitioners' preference to administer methylergonovine directly into the uterine corpus.[20] However, it has been reported that inappropriate myometrial absorption of methylergonovine was a suspected cause of myocardial ischemia, likely because the highly vascularized myometrial tissue increased the rate of systemic uptake.[28] Due to the potential for hypertensive or cerebrovascular events, intravenous injection is not recommended. If intravenous administration of methylergonovine is necessary as a lifesaving measure, it should be given slowly over a period of more than 60 seconds with close blood pressure monitoring. Methylergonovine also can be given orally for up to 1 week.[21]

Side Effects and Contraindications

The most common negative side effect of methylergonovine is hypertension due to vasoconstriction. This can be associated with headaches or seizures.[21] Methylergonovine has rarely been associated with coronary vasospasm, myocardial ischemia, and myocardial infarction. Patients with coronary artery disease or risk factors for coronary artery disease are at increased risk of developing acute coronary syndrome or infarction. These risk factors include smoking, obesity, diabetes, and high cholesterol. In a large retrospective study, no significant increase in myocardial ischemia or infarction was seen with methylergonovine administration. Of the patients with chronic ischemic heart disease or risk factors for heart disease, only 1 case of myocardial ischemia/infarction was found out of 14,489 patients who received methylergonovine.[29] ACOG recommends avoiding methylergonovine in hypertensive patients. Nausea and vomiting also have been reported. Other rare adverse reactions include bradycardia, tachycardia, hypotension, dyspnea, thrombophlebitis, dizziness, and diarrhea.[21]

Methylergonovine goes through CYP3A4 metabolism. Potent CYP3A4 inhibitors (such as protease inhibitors, erythromycin, quinolones, ketoconazole) should be avoided. Other ergot alkaloids or vasoconstrictors must be used with extreme caution when coadministered. Other contraindications include sepsis, pregnancy, and hypersensitivity.[21]

Summary and Discussion

Methylergonovine is recommended by ACOG and the Royal College of Obstetrics and Gynecology as a second-line uterotonic. However, no recommendations are made regarding the choice of a specific second-line agent. A recent study using a nationwide dataset found that the frequency of second-line uterotonics use was 7.1%. Methylergonovine was used at a frequency of 5.2%, carboprost at 1.0%, and misoprostol at 1.2%.[30] Methylergonovine has been shown to decrease the amount of postpartum hemorrhage–related morbidity and reduced the amount to a greater extent than carboprost.[26] Although recent safety concerns about methylergonovine-induced vasoconstriction causing myocardial ischemia and infarction have been reported, the risk is exceedingly low. For a patient with no history or risk factors for coronary disease, methylergonovine is an extremely effective agent to correct refractory uterine atony and mitigate the postpartum hemorrhage.

CARBOPROST

Introduction

Carboprost (US brand name Hemabate) is an analog of prostaglandin F2α. Maternal concentrations of endogenous prostaglandins increase during labor, with peak concentrations occurring at the time of placental separation. This prostaglandin surge likely contributes to uterine contractions and placental delivery. One cause of uterine atony may be a deficiency of prostaglandin F2α concentration increase during the third stage of labor.[31,32]

Structure/Activity

Rapid metabolism of naturally occurring prostaglandins limited their usefulness for clinical application and led to the development of analogs with longer durations of action. Carboprost tromethamine, the active ingredient in Hemabate, is an analog of 15-methyl prostaglandin F2α. Naturally occurring prostaglandins are oxidized at carbon 15, which causes rapid inactivation of primary prostaglandins. On the analog, this oxidation is completely blocked, with the hydrogen being replaced by a methyl group.[33]

Myometrial intracellular free calcium concentration is increased by prostaglandins. The increased availability of calcium leads to increased myosin light-chain kinase activity, augmenting the contractile response of the uterus.[34,35]

Pharmacokinetics

Carboprost is injected intramuscularly for the treatment of postpartum hemorrhage. Plasma levels peak 20 minutes after injection, and decline by approximately half after 2 hours.[33]

Urinary excretion is the major route of elimination of carboprost. Excretion of metabolites is almost complete 24 hours after subcutaneous administration in women. Approximately 80% of the dose is excreted within the first 5 to 10 hours, with an additional 5% of the dose excreted over the next 20 hours. Three major metabolites of carboprost have been identified in human urine. Approximately 1% of the dose is excreted as intact drug.[36]

Clinical Role

Carboprost is a second-line treatment for uterine atony. Most cases of uterine atony respond to manual uterine massage and oxytocin. For refractory uterine atony with or without postpartum hemorrhage, both methylergonovine and carboprost are used in an effort to avoid surgical interventions such as ligation of the uterine or hypogastric arteries or peripartum hysterectomy. Methylergonovine is associated with a lowered risk of hemorrhage-related morbidity during cesarean delivery when compared with carboprost. Women receiving carboprost were 1.7 times as likely to have hemorrhage-related morbidity.[26] Carboprost is a treatment alternative for patients with hypertensive disorders, such as preeclampsia (a relative contraindication to methylergonovine), and for patients with atonic bleeding refractory to methylergonovine.[34,37]

Routes and Dosage

Carboprost for uterine atony should be administered intramuscularly. The recommended dose is 250 μg. The dosage may be repeated every 15 to 30 minutes. Total dose should not exceed 2 mg (8 dosages). In clinical trials, 80% of patients with uterine atony responded to less than 250 μg and 95% of patients responded to less than 500 μg.[36,38] For women with severe postpartum hemorrhage who had already failed conventional therapy with intravenous oxytocin, intramuscular methylergonovine and manual uterine massage, studies showed a rescue rate of 86% overall, with 88% of subjects responding after 2 intramuscular doses.[34] The need for repeated doses should be evaluated based on clinical effect.

Side Effects and Contraindications

Frequently reported side effects of carboprost administration include nausea, vomiting, and diarrhea. The cause of these adverse effects is likely the stimulation of smooth muscle in the gastrointestinal tract. Flushing, pyrexia, and myalgia are also reported. Moderate increases in blood pressure are often seen, caused by vascular smooth muscle contraction.[36] The observed effect on blood pressure is clinically insignificant when compared with the effect of methylergonovine.

Carboprost can precipitate bronchospasm, increased intrapulmonary shunt fraction, abnormal ventilation-perfusion ratio, and hypoxemia. Patients with asthma are particularly susceptible to these complications, but there are rare documented cases of bronchospasm in patients without asthma.[38–41] In asthmatic patients, the resulting bronchospasm can be severe and can occur after only 1 dose.

The use of carboprost in breastfeeding mothers has not been specifically studied, but based on plasma clearance rates, the manufacturer recommends that breastfeeding be delayed for at least 6 hours after administration.[36]

Summary and Discussion

Carboprost, an analog of prostaglandin F2α, has an important role in the management of refractory uterine atony. When first-line treatment with manual uterine massage and oxytocin has failed, and methylergonovine is contraindicated or has not been effective, it is imperative that uterine tone be restored to prevent life-threatening postpartum hemorrhage. Carboprost is successful in triggering uterine smooth muscle contraction after the first or second dose in approximately 90% of cases. Although the mechanism of action can lead to unpleasant side effects, such as vomiting or diarrhea, these issues are minor when compared with the risks associated with major hemorrhage, massive transfusion, or surgical intervention. The only relative contraindication to the use of carboprost is asthma. Asthmatic patients can experience life-threatening bronchospasm after a single dose of carboprost.

MISOPROSTOL

Introduction

Misoprostol, a synthetic analog of prostaglandin E1, has a long history of medical application. Naturally occurring prostaglandin E1 (PGE1) protects gastric mucosa through reduction in gastric acid secretion and stimulation of mucus and bicarbonate secretion. Originally developed as a treatment for peptic ulcers, misoprostol found a vital role in obstetric and gynecologic patients thanks to its effects on uterine smooth muscle and the cervix. The list of clinical applications has since grown to include medically induced abortion, medically assisted evacuation after miscarriage, cervical ripening, induction of labor, and treatment of uterine atony.

Structure/Activity

Misoprostol is a synthetic prostaglandin E1 analog (15-deoxy-16-hydroxy-16-methyl PGE1). Compared with PGE1, misoprostol exhibits superior performance across 3 notable areas. PGE1 is rapidly metabolized, which hinders its utility via oral and parenteral routes, and it also produces more side effects while being less chemically stable. PGE1 has a carboxyl group at carbon 1 and a hydroxyl group at carbon 15. Misoprostol improves on the characteristics of PGE1 by having a methyl ester at carbon 1 (imparting greater duration of action), a carbon 16 methyl group, and hydroxyl group at carbon 16 rather than carbon 15. The modifications at carbon 16 increase oral activity, duration of action, and safety.[42]

Pharmacokinetics

Misoprostol has differing pharmacokinetic profiles depending on the route of administration, and clinically useful routes include the following: oral, buccal, sublingual, vaginal, and rectal. In terms of speed of onset, the oral and sublingual routes appear to be superior. Sublingual administration yields the highest peak plasma concentrations of any route, and peak plasma concentrations are seen in approximately 30 minutes.[43] Concomitant food intake and antacid use will measurably reduce the availability of oral misoprostol, but it is not clear whether the effect is clinically significant.[44]

Vaginal administrations of misoprostol produce slower onset and a longer time to peak effect than routes involving the mouth; however, the decline in plasma concentration is also much slower, with corresponding superiority in terms of bioavailability. Vaginal absorption can vary significantly with the vaginal environment, where pH changes and varying amounts of vaginal discharge can potentially alter the observed pharmacokinetics.[45] In the context of vaginal bleeding from uterine atony or medical abortion, vaginal absorption may be reduced.

Buccal misoprostol exhibits a time to peak concentration and a gradual fall in concentration comparable to the kinetics of vaginal misoprostol, but with inferior bioavailability to both sublingual and vaginal routes.[46,47]

Rectal misoprostol generates the slowest onset, with a long offset time comparable to that of vaginal misoprostol.[48] Serum concentrations, reflecting bioavailability after rectal administration, remain inferior to levels seen after vaginal misoprostol.[46]

Misoprostol exhibits extensive renal clearance, and renal impairment may extend its half-life as well as increase bioavailability and maximum plasma concentrations. However, there is no recommended dose adjustment for patients in renal failure.[44]

Misoprostol acid is found in breast milk for several hours after oral administration, albeit in concentrations lower than maternal serum concentrations.[49,50] The FDA warns that nursing mothers may cause significant diarrhea in their infants by breastfeeding under these circumstances.[44]

Clinical Role

Misoprostol is a second-line agent for treatment of uterine atony. During and after the third stage of labor, oxytocin is the first-line agent given to all patients to prevent postpartum hemorrhage. In situations in which oxytocin is not immediately available, or when oxytocin fails to produce a desired result, methylergonovine has advantages of speed and efficacy over misoprostol. However, in patients with a contraindication to methylergonovine therapy, or in environments in which skilled attendants and supplies are not available to deliver injectable medications, or if methylergonovine is not immediately available, misoprostol can be used.[51] In medically underserved areas where the supply and storage of expensive, or light-sensitive or temperature-sensitive medications is limited, misoprostol tablets offer an inexpensive and easy-to-store uterotonic option.[52] Misoprostol also can be given to patients whose uterine atony is refractory to earlier interventions,[53] but in a major meta-analysis there was no clear benefit to using misoprostol as an adjuvant to oxytocin in terms of major outcomes, such as mortality and blood loss.[54]

In a meta-analysis of recent large randomized controlled trials involving misoprostol versus placebo, misoprostol effectively prevented postpartum hemorrhage and severe postpartum hemorrhage by 24% and 41%, respectively.[55]

Routes and Dosage

Numerous studies have evaluated the optimal route and dose for misoprostol in postpartum hemorrhage applications. As a first-line treatment in situations in which active management of the third stage of labor is not possible, 800 μg has the most evidence supporting its safety and efficacy as a single sublingual dose.[54] For postpartum hemorrhage, 600 μg has been advocated as an oral or sublingual treatment dose[53] and this is also a well-studied prophylactic dose.[55] A 600-μg oral dose of misoprostol begins to act within 3 to 5 minutes.[51] However, oral doses of 400 to 600 μg do not appear to have differing clinical efficacy, whereas the larger dose is associated with a greater incidence of pyrexia.[56,57] Repeat doses of misoprostol are not recommended for at least 2 hours, or 6 hours in patients exhibiting shivering and pyrexia.[53]

Vaginal administration of misoprostol may not be practical during active postpartum hemorrhage with vaginal bleeding. Rectal administration has been studied, but that route is not recommended for treatment or prevention of atonic uterine bleeding.

Side Effects and Contraindications

Misoprostol has no serious side effects in doses and durations of therapy that are clinically appropriate for the treatment of uterine atony. If misoprostol is effective in eliciting uterine contractions, patients may complain of cramping. Gastrointestinal upset may occur. With increasing doses, misoprostol has been described to cause shivering and corresponding hyperthermia.[58] Side effects are self-limited and may be more common with sublingual misoprostol administration due to its pharmacokinetics, notably the high peak serum concentrations that correspond to that route.[47]

The toxic dose of misoprostol is not known. A dose of 1600 μg in a single day has been tolerated in patients but may cause gastrointestinal upset. Overdose may produce symptoms including sedation, tremor, convulsions, dyspnea, abdominal pain, diarrhea, fever, palpitations, hypotension, or bradycardia. Treatment for overdose is supportive, as there is no known reversal agent and dialysis is unlikely to help clear misoprostol acid, the detectable and biologically active form of misoprostol.[44]

There are no contraindications to using misoprostol in postpartum patients other than history of an allergic reaction.[53] The only FDA warning related to misoprostol applies to pregnant or potentially pregnant women due to its abortifacient and possible teratogenic effects.[44]

Summary and Discussion

Misoprostol has a role in the management of uterine atony. Because of its wide variety of clinical applications, misoprostol is an active topic of research. Questions remain about the optimal dose and route, and whether prophylactic use should be limited to situations in which active management of the third stage of labor (eg, oxytocin) is not possible. But its ease of administration, modest side-effect profile, lack of contraindications, and proven efficacy make it a useful option.

SUMMARY

Conditions that increase the risk of uterine atony, such as overdistention of the uterus (as seen with multiple gestations and polyhydramnios), magnesium sulfate administrations and chorioamnionitis are frequently encountered in clinical practice. With the incidence of postpartum hemorrhage increasing and with uterine atony a contributor in many cases, it is important to understand the risks and benefits of commonly used uterotonic agents.[59] Manual uterine massage and oxytocin are almost universally accepted as the first-line treatments of choice for uterine atony. When this combination is ineffective, it is often appropriate to administer a second-line uterotonic agent. Methylergonovine and carboprost are second-line agents in most treatment protocols. The choice of which therapeutic agent to use should be based on the comorbidities of the patient and the clinical judgment of the practitioners involved in the case. Misoprostol remains a treatment option for uterine atony, but its utility as an adjunct to the other uterotonic medications may be limited.

REFERENCES

1. Dale HH. The action of extracts of the pituitary body. Biochem J 1909;4:427–47.
2. Du Vigneaud V, Ressler C, Swan JM, et al. Oxytocin: synthesis. J Am Chem Soc 1954;76(12):3115–8.

3. Gimpl G, Fahrenholz F. The oxytocin receptor system: structure, function, and regulation. Physiol Rev 2001;81:629–83.
4. Dyer RA, Van Dyk D, Dresner A. The use of uterotonic drugs during caesarean section. Int J Obstet Anesth 2010;19:313–9.
5. Arais F. Pharmacology of oxytocin and prostaglandins. Clin Obstet Gynecol 2000; 43:455–68.
6. Dyer RA, Butwick AJ, Carvalho B. Oxytocin for labour caesarean delivery: implications for the the anaesthesiologist. Curr Opin Anesthesiol 2011;24:255–61.
7. Oladapo OT, Okusanya BO, Abalos E. Intramuscular versus intravenous prophylactic oxytocin for the third sate of labour. Cochrane Database Syst Rev 2012;(2):CD009332.
8. Dawood MY, Ylikorkala O, Trivedi D, et al. Oxytocin levels and disappearance rate and plasma follicle-stimulant hormone and luteinizing hormone after oxytocin infusion in men. J Clin Endocrinol Metab 1980;50:397–400.
9. Seitchik J, Amico J, Robinson AG, et al. Oxytocin augmentation of dysfunctional labor. IV. Oxytocin pharmacokinetics. Am J Obstet Gynecol 1984;150:225–8.
10. Mitchell BF, Feng X, Wong S. Oxytocin: a paracrine hormone in the regulation of parturition? Rev Reprod 1998;3:113–22.
11. Thomas JS, Koh SH, Cooper GM. Haemodynamic effects of oxytocin given as IV bolus or infusion on women undergoing caesarean section. Br J Anaesth 2007; 98(1):116–9.
12. Carvalho JC, Balki M, Kingdom J, et al. Oxytocin requirements at elective cesarean delivery: a dose-finding study. Obstet Gynecol 2004;104:10005–10.
13. Balki M, Ronayane M, Davies S, et al. Minimum oxytocin dose requirement after cesarean delivery for labor arrest. Obstet Gynecol 2006;104:45–50.
14. Kimura T, Tanizawa O, Mori K, et al. Structure and expression of a human oxytocin receptor. Nature 1992;356:526–9.
15. Phaneuf S, Rodriguez LB, TambyRaja RL, et al. Loss of myometrial oxytocin receptors during oxytocin-induced and oxytocin-augmented labour. J Reprod Fertil 2000;120:91–7.
16. Kovacheva FP, Soens MA, Tsen LC. A randomized, double-blinded trial of a "rule of threes" algorithm versus continuous infusion of oxytocin during elective cesarean delivery. Anesthesiology 2015;123(1):92–9.
17. Pinder AJ, Dresner C, Calow C, et al. Haemodynamic changes caused by oxytocin during caesarean section under spinal anesthesia. Int J Obstet Anesth 2002;11:156–9.
18. Begrum D, Lonnee H, Hakli TF. Oxytocin infusion: acute hyponatremia, seizures, and coma. Acta Anasthesiol Scand 2009;53:826–7.
19. de Groot AN, van Dongen PW, Vree TB, et al. Ergot alkaloids. Current status and review of clinical pharmacology and therapeutic use compared with other oxytocics in obstetrics and gynaecology. Drugs 1998;56(4):523–35.
20. American College of Obstetricians and Gynecologists. ACOG Practice Bulletin: Clinical Management Guidelines for Obstetrician-Gynecologists Number 76, October 2006: postpartum hemorrhage. Obstet Gynecol 2006;108(4):1039–47.
21. Novartis. Methergine (methylergonovine maleate). Injection Label. U.S. Food and Drug Adminstration. 2012. Available at: http://www.accessdata.fda.gov/drugsatfda_docs/label/2012/006035s078lbl.pdf. Accessed August 31, 2016.
22. Schiff PL. Ergot and its alkaloids. Am J Pharm Educ 2006;70(5):98.
23. de Groot AN. The role of oral (methyl)ergometrine in the prevention of postpartum haemorrhage. Eur J Obstet Gynecol Reprod Biol 1996;69(1):31–6.

24. Gao Y, Sun Q, Liu D, et al. A sensitive LC-MS/MS method to quantify methylergonovine in human plasma and its application to a pharmacokinetic study. J Chromatogr B Analyt Technol Biomed Life Sci 2016;1011:62–8.
25. Gizzo S, Patrelli TS, Gangi SD, et al. Which uterotonic is better to prevent the postpartum hemorrhage? Latest news in terms of clinical efficacy, side effects, and contraindications: a systematic review. Reprod Sci 2013;20(9):1011–9.
26. Butwick AJ, Carvalho B, Blumenfeld YJ, et al. Second-line uterotonics and the risk of hemorrhage-related morbidity. Am J Obstet Gynecol 2015;212:642.e1-7.
27. Saper JR, Evans RW. Oral methylergonovine maleate for refractory migraine and cluster headache prevention. Headache 2013;53(2):378–81.
28. Kuczkowski KM. Myocardial ischemia induced by intramyometrial injection of methylergonovine maleate. Anesthesiology 2004;100(4):1043.
29. Bateman BT, Huybrechts KF, Hernandez-Diaz S, et al. Methylergonovine maleate and the risk of myocardial ischemia and infarction. Am J Obstet Gynecol 2013; 209(5):459.e1–13.
30. Bateman BT, Tsen LC, Liu J, et al. Patterns of second-line uterotonic use in a large sample of hospitalizations for childbirth in the United States: 2007-2011. Anesth Analg 2014;119(6):1344–9.
31. Noort WA, van Bulck B, Vereecken A, et al. Changes in plasma levels of PGF2α and PGI2 metabolites at and after delivery at term. Prostaglandins 1989;37:3–12.
32. Fuchs AR, Husslein P, Sumulong L, et al. The origin of circulating 13,14-dihydro-15-keto-prostaglandin F2α during delivery. Prostaglandins 1982;24:715–22.
33. Bygdeman M. Pharmacokinetics of prostaglandins. Best Pract Res Clin Obstet Gynaecol 2003;17:707–16.
34. Hayashi RH, Castillo MS, Noah ML. Management of severe postpartum hemorrhage with a prostaglandin F2α analogue. Obstet Gynecol 1984;63:806–8.
35. Izumi H, Garfield RE, Morishita F, et al. Some mechanical properties of skinned fibres of pregnant human myometrium. Eur J Obstet Gynecol Reprod Biol 1994;56:55–62.
36. Pfizer. Hemabate (carboprost tromethamine). U.S. Food and Drug Administration. 2013. Available at: http://www.accessdata.fda.gov/drugsatfda_docs/label/2013/017989s019lbl.pdf. Accessed August 22, 2016.
37. Bigrigg A, Chissell S, Read MD. Use of intra myometrial 15-methyl prostaglandin F2α to control atonic postpartum haemorrhage following vaginal delivery and failure of conventional therapy. Br J Obstet Gynaecol 1991;98:734–6.
38. O'Leary AM. Severe bronchospasm and hypotension after 15-methyl prostaglandin F2α in atonic postpartum haemorrhage. Int J Obstet Anesth 1994;3:42–4.
39. Andersen LH, Secher NJ. Pattern of total and regional lung function in subjects with bronchoconstriction induced by 15-methyl PGF2α. Thorax 1976;31:685–92.
40. Cooley DM, Glosten B, Roberts JR, et al. Bronchospasm after intramuscular 15-methyl prostaglandin F sub 2 alpha, 125 micrograms, and intravenous oxytocin, 20 units, for the control of blood loss at elective cesarean section. Am J Obstet Gynecol 1994;171:1356–60.
41. Harper C, Levy D, Chidambaram S, et al. Life-threatening bronchospasm after intramuscular carboprost for postpartum hemorrhage. BJOG 2007;114:366–8.
42. Tang OS, Gemzell-Danielsson K, Ho PC. Misoprostol. Pharmacokinetic profiles, effects on the uterus, and side-effects. Int J Gynecol Obstet 2007;99:S160–7.
43. Tang OS, Schweer H, Seyberth HW, et al. Pharmacokinetics of different routes of administration of misoprostol. Hum Reprod 2002;17:332–6.

44. GD Searle & Co. Cytotec® (misoprostol). U.S. Food and Drug Administration. 2002. Available at: http://www.accessdata.fda.gov/drugsatfda_docs/label/2002/19268slr037.pdf. Accessed August 12, 2016.
45. Zieman M, Fong SK, Benowitz NL, et al. Absorption kinetics of misoprostol with oral or vaginal administration. Obstet Gynecol 1997;90:88–92.
46. Meckstroth KR, Whitaker AK, Bertisch S, et al. Misoprostol administered by epithelial routes. Obstet Gynecol 2006;108:82–90.
47. Schaff EA, DiCenzo R, Fielding SL. Comparison of misoprostol plasma concentrations following buccal and sublingual administration. Contraception 2005;71:22–5.
48. Khan RU, El-Refaey H. Pharmacokinetics and adverse-effect profile of rectally administered misoprostol in the third stage of labor. Obstet Gynecol 2003;101:968–74.
49. Abdel-Aleem H, Villar J, Gulmezoglu AM, et al. The pharmacokinetics of the prostaglandin E1 analogue misoprostol in plasma and colostrum after postpartum oral administration. Eur J Obstet Gynecol Reprod Biol 2003;108:25–8.
50. Vogel D, Burkhardt T, Rentsch K, et al. Misoprostol versus methylergometrine: pharmacokinetics in human milk. Am J Obstet Gynecol 2004;191:2168–73.
51. POPPHI. Fact sheets: uterotonic drugs for the prevention and treatment of postpartum hemorrhage. Seattle (WA): PATH; 2008.
52. McCormick ML, Sanghvi HC, Kinzie B, et al. Preventing postpartum hemorrhage in low-resource settings. Int J Gynaecol Obstet 2002;77:267–75.
53. Blum J, Alfirevic Z, Walraven G, et al. Treatment of postpartum hemorrhage with misoprostol. Int J Gynaecol Obstet 2007;99(Suppl 2):S202–5.
54. Mousa HA, Blum J, Abou EL, et al. Treatment for primary postpartum hemorrhage. Cochrane Database Syst Rev 2014;(2):CD003249.
55. Oladapo OT. Misoprostol for preventing and treating postpartum hemorrhage in the community: a closer look at the evidence. Int J Gynaecol Obstet 2012;119:105–10.
56. Hofmeyr J, Gulmezolgu AM, Novikova N, et al. Misoprostol to prevent and treat postpartum haemorrhage: a systematic review and meta-analysis of maternal deaths and dose-related effects. Bull World Health Organ 2009;87:666–77.
57. Hofmeyr GJ, Gulmezoglu AM, Novikova N, et al. Postpartum misoprostol for preventing maternal mortality and morbidity. Cochrane Database Syst Rev 2013;(7):CD008982.
58. Lumbiganon P, Hofmeyr J, Gulmezoglu AM, et al. Misoprostol dose-related shivering and pyrexia in the third stage of labour. WHO Collaborative Trial of Misoprostol in the Management of the Third Stage of Labour. BJOG 1999;106:304–8.
59. Bateman BT, Berman MF, Riley LE, et al. The epidemiology of postpartum hemorrhage in a large, nationwide sample of deliveries. Anesth Analg 2010;110(5):1368–73.

Pulmonary Vasodilators and Anesthesia Considerations

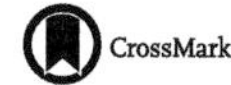

Jeremy B. Green, MD[a], Brendon Hart, DO[b], Elyse M. Cornett, PhD[b], Alan D. Kaye, MD, PhD, DABA, DABPM, DABIPP[c,*], Ali Salehi, MD[d], Charles J. Fox, MD[b]

KEYWORDS

• Pulmonary hypertension • Anesthesia • Inhaled nitric oxide • Endothelin antagonists • Calcium channel blockers • Prostacyclin

KEY POINTS

- The normal adult pulmonary circulation is a low-pressure, low-resistance circuit that accommodates the whole output of the right ventricle to the gas exchanging surface at less than one-fifth of systemic pressure.
- Vasodilators normally have little if any effect on pulmonary vascular pressures, indicating that there is little or no resting tone under healthy conditions.
- Factors including the autonomic nervous system, humoral agents, and atmospheric gases, have the ability to alter pulmonary vascular resistance by inducing contraction or relaxation of vascular smooth muscle in resistance vessels elements in the lung.
- There are three major underlying components involved in the pathogenesis of pulmonary arterial hypertension: endothelial dysfunction leading to vasoconstriction, vascular remodeling with in situ thrombosis, and the formation of plexiform lesions.
- Numerous pulmonary vasodilators are currently being evaluated and being used in the treatment of pulmonary hypertension, including calcium channel blockers, inhaled nitric oxide, prostacyclin derivatives, endothelin antagonists, phosphodiesterase (PDE)-5 inhibitors, and diuretics.

INTRODUCTION

Pulmonary hypertension (PH) is a complex disease process of the pulmonary vasculature system characterized by elevated pulmonary arterial pressures (PAP). Despite being a rare disease, patients with PH represent a distinct challenge in the operating

[a] Department of Anesthesiology, Louisiana State University Health Science Center-New Orleans, New Orleans, LA, USA; [b] Department of Anesthesiology, Louisiana State University Health Science Center-Shreveport, Shreveport, LA, USA; [c] Department of Anesthesiology, Louisiana State University Health Science Center-New Orleans, 1542 Tulane Avenue, New Orleans, LA 70112, USA; [d] Department of Anesthesiology, Ronald Regan UCLA Medical Center, Los Angeles, CA, USA
* Corresponding author.
E-mail address: alankaye44@hotmail.com

Anesthesiology Clin 35 (2017) 221–232
http://dx.doi.org/10.1016/j.anclin.2017.01.008
anesthesiology.theclinics.com
1932-2275/17/

room given their increased risks for morbidity and mortality, even in the setting of noncardiac surgeries. Studies suggest that the postoperative mortality rate for patients with PH ranges from 1% to 18%,[1] whereas perioperative morbidity rates may be 42% and include complications, such as respiratory failure, dysrhythmias, congestive heart failure, renal insufficiency, hemodynamic instability, hepatic dysfunction, myocardial infarction, and even stroke.[2]

Over the past two decades, the classification system for PH has undergone several changes, with the most recent update coming in 2013 following the 5th World Symposium on Pulmonary Hypertension. Previously divided into primary pulmonary hypertension (no identifiable cause) and secondary pulmonary hypertension (identifiable cause), it is now divided into five different groups based on several specific etiologies (**Box 1**):

- Group 1: Pulmonary arterial hypertension
- Group 2: PH caused by left heart disease
- Group 3: PH caused by chronic lung disease and/or hypoxemia
- Group 4: Chronic thromboembolic PH
- Group 5: PH caused by unclear multifactorial mechanisms

PH is defined by a mean PAP greater than or equal to 25 mm Hg at rest via right heart catheterization, whereas the category 1 (pulmonary arterial hypertension [PAH]) also requires a pulmonary artery wedge pressure equal to less than 15 and a pulmonary vascular resistance (PVR) greater than 3 woods units.

Related to a multitude of causes, and the insidious onset of PH, prevalence data in the general population are unclear. One individual study used national registries to examine mortality rates for patients with all types of PH and found that African Americans were most affected (7.3 per 100,000), followed by females (5.5 per 100,000), males (5.4 per 100,000), and white persons (5.3 per 100,000).[3]

Further studies have focused on data for PAH, which includes idiopathic and heritable causes of PH. Research using national registries from the United Kingdom and Ireland showed an incidence of 1.1 cases per million each year with and overall prevalence of 6.6 cases per million.[4] Similar studies from France showed an incidence and prevalence of 2.4 cases per million annually and 15 cases per million, respectively.[5]

Traditionally, PAH was thought to be a disease of middle-aged women. More recent registries, however, have shown an increase in the mean age at diagnosis up from 36 $\pm$ 15 years (1981[6]) to between 50 $\pm$ 14 and 65 $\pm$ 15 years[7] and a female-to-male ratio of 1.2:1 among the elderly.[8]

Although there is no cure for PAH, multiple meta-analyses have shown decreases in morbidity and mortality thanks to the development of prostacyclins, endothelin antagonists, and phosphodiesterase (PDE)-5 inhibitors.[9,10] Still, 1-year mortality rate remains high at 15%.[11]

STRUCTURE OF PULMONARY VESSELS AND THE ROLE OF ENDOTHELIUM AND NEURAL MECHANISMS

Pulmonary arteries, in contrast to systemic arteries, have a much thinner smooth muscle layer under normal physiologic states. Small pulmonary arteries of several hundred micrometers internal diameter are the major site of vascular resistance and are the site of hypoxic pulmonary vasoconstriction.[12] The pulmonary capillary bed is the major site of action and metabolism of several vasoactive agents. Pulmonary veins are similar in structure to pulmonary arteries but have less smooth muscle

Box 1
Classification of pulmonary hypertension

1. Pulmonary arterial hypertension
   - 1.1. Idiopathic pulmonary arterial hypertension
   - 1.2. Heritable pulmonary arterial hypertension
     - 1.2.1. BMPR2
     - 1.2.2. ALK1, ENG, SMAD9, CAV1, KCNK3
     - 1.2.3. Unknown
   - 1.3. Drug- and toxin-induced
   - 1.4. Associated with
     - 1.4.1. Connective tissue diseases
     - 1.4.2. Human immunodeficiency virus infection
     - 1.4.3. Portal hypertension
     - 1.4.4. Congenital heart disease
     - 1.4.5. Schistosomiasis
   - 1′. Pulmonary veno-occlusive disease and/or pulmonary capillary hemangiomatosis
   - 1″. Persistent pulmonary hypertension of the newborn
2. Pulmonary hypertension caused by left heart disease
   - 2.1. Left ventricular systolic dysfunction
   - 2.2. Left ventricular diastolic dysfunction
   - 2.3. Valvular disease
   - 2.4. Congenital/acquired left heart inflow/outflow tract obstruction and congenital cardiomyopathies
3. Pulmonary hypertension caused by lung diseases and/or hypoxia
   - 3.1. Chronic obstructive pulmonary disease
   - 3.2. Interstitial lung disease
   - 3.3. Other pulmonary diseases with mixed restrictive and obstructive pattern
   - 3.4. Sleep-disordered breathing
   - 3.5. Alveolar hypoventilation disorders
   - 3.6. Chronic exposure to high altitude
   - 3.7. Developmental lung diseases
4. Chronic thromboembolic pulmonary hypertension
5. Pulmonary hypertension with unclear multifactorial mechanisms
   - 5.1. Hematologic disorders: chronic hemolytic anemia, myeloproliferative disorders, splenectomy
   - 5.2. Systemic disorders: sarcoidosis, pulmonary histiocytosis, lymphangioleiomyomatosis
   - 5.3. Metabolic disorders: glycogen storage disease, Gaucher disease, thyroid disorders
   - 5.4. Others: tumoral obstruction, fibrosing mediastinitis, chronic renal failure, segmental pulmonary hypertension

From Simonneau G, Robbins IM, Beghetti M. Updated clinical classification of pulmonary hypertension. J Am Coll Cardiol 2009;54(1):S45; with permission.

and may have different receptors. Constriction of pulmonary arteries results in elevated PAP, which increases the pressure on the right side of the heart, whereas constriction of pulmonary veins increases pulmonary capillary pressure, which could result in pulmonary edema. In many pathophysiologic processes, the structure of pulmonary vessels may change dramatically. With a chronic increase in pulmonary vascular pressure, there is a structural remodeling with fibrosis, particularly in the intimal layer, and increased size of the smooth muscle layer. This may result in a marked alteration in function.

In this regard, endothelial cells in the pulmonary circulation have a profound influence on vascular tone. Endothelial cells have the capacity to release several constrictor and dilator substances, and agents that affect the growth and differentiation of cells in the vessel wall.[13] Many agents influence pulmonary vascular tone via the release of endothelial mediators. Modulation of angiotensin peptide responses has been demonstrated with endothelial lining removal.[14] It has been hypothesized that the release of endothelial-derived nitric oxide (NO) may serve to modulate the vasoconstrictor effects of endogenous agonists, such as the angiotensin peptides. The autonomic nervous system may modify pulmonary blood flow distribution under physiologic conditions and may be involved in pathophysiologic states. Pulmonary vascular tone is regulated by many autonomic receptors. Ultrastructural studies have confirmed not only the existence of adrenergic nerve profiles, but in addition, cholinergic innervation in the pulmonary arteries of many species, including the cat.[15]

Although it is well-established that endothelial cells play a key role in the formation of angiotensin II from angiotensin I, because of the presence of angiotensin I–converting enzyme on the plasma membrane, endothelial cells may also possess an endogenous renin-angiotensin system.[16] Incubation of 12^5 I-angiotensin-I with bovine and human endothelial cells resulted in the production of larger amounts of hepapeptide angiotensin-(1–7) (Asp-Arg-Val-Tyr-Ile-His-Pro) than of the octapeptide angiotensin II.[17] When the cells were treated with the angiotensin I–converting enzyme inhibitor enalaprilat, the production of angiotensin 1 to 7 increased, suggesting that human endothelium possesses a metabolic route independent of angiotensin-converting enzyme for the processing of angiotensin I.

PATHOPHYSIOLOGY

Compared with the systemic circulatory system, the pulmonary vasculature system is characterized by low pressure, typically about one-fifth of systemic pressure, and low resistance, related in part to a thinner media and the absence of muscular arterioles. This allows it to accommodate large amounts of blood volume despite a small pressure gradient.[18] There are several factors that regulate PVR to direct blood flow to particular parts of the lung, the most important being oxygenation. Contrary to the systemic circulation, which dilates in response to hypoxia, pulmonary vasculature undergoes hypoxic vasoconstriction to optimize ventilation-perfusion matching. Minor increases in PVR have been noted with Po_2 levels less than 60 mm Hg, with more significant responses seen as Po_2 approaches 45 mm Hg.[19] Other influences on PVR include pulmonary blood flow, lung volume, CO^2 levels, PH, pulmonary vascular endothelium, and vascular mediators.[20–22]

Although CO_2 does not have a direct effect on the vascular endothelium, hypercapnia leads to acidosis and a reflexive increase in PVR and is thought to assist the role of hypoxic pulmonary vasoconstriction.[23]

As cardiac output increases, blood flow increases via recruitment of previously closed vessels within the lung and via dilation of previously opened vessels. Recruitment of further vessels leads to an increase in area of flow, inversely decreasing the PVR.

The relationship between lung volume and PVR is uniquely represented by a U-shaped curve, with PVR increased at high and low lung volumes, whereas PVR is lowest at the functional residual capacity. At low lung volumes PVR is elevated because of decreased tension in extra-alveolar arterioles, whereas at high volumes the PVR is elevated because of compression of alveolar capillaries.[18]

Vascular endothelium is capable of decreasing PVR via two major pathways. O^2, shear force, ATP, and vascular endothelial growth factor activate the enzymes NO synthase and cyclooxygenase, which leads to the subsequent production of NO and prostacyclin. NO and Prostaglandin I2 (PGI2) work at the level of smooth muscle to increase the levels of cGMP and cAMP, respectively, both of which lead to relaxation and vasodilation.

There are three major underlying components involved in the pathogenesis of PAH: (1) endothelial dysfunction leading to vasoconstriction, (2) vascular remodeling with in situ thrombosis, and (3) the formation of plexiform lesions.

In the simplest sense, PH is caused by a prolonged increase in PVR. An imbalance in endothelial-derived factors leads to increased activity of thromboxane and endothelin (vasoconstrictors) coupled with a decrease in local vasodilators NO and PGI2. In addition to vasoconstriction, this imbalance also leads to stimulation of smooth muscle and subsequent platelet aggregation.[18] Increased levels of serotonin have also been shown to decrease the ratio of vasodilators to vasoconstrictors.[24] Chronic vasoconstriction and hypoxemia seen with worsening disease lead to the proliferation of endothelial and smooth muscle cells.[25] Loss of function mutation in the bone morphogenic protein-2 receptor has been recognized as playing a role in the development of heritable PAH. Normally involved with growth inhibition and proapoptotic signaling of smooth muscle cells, loss of function of the receptor may lead to further proliferation.[26–28] Dysregulation of vascular remodeling leads to intimal thickening and a subsequent increase in PVR.[29] Additionally, levels of thrombogenic factors are known to be elevated in PH.[30,31] A hallmark of late-stage PH is the histologic formation of plexiform lesions, or complex vascular formations that are seen from the remodeling and obliteration of pulmonary arteries.[18]

CRITERIA AND DIAGNOSIS OF PULMONARY HYPERTENSION

Because the initial symptoms of PH are so nonspecific, early diagnosis of the disease has proved challenging for clinicians. Dyspnea on exertion, lethargy, and fatigue are often misattributed to old age or other comorbid conditions, allowing for further progression of the disease. Often it is not until the disease has advanced to later stages that PH is diagnosed. A study by Brown and colleagues[32] showed that 21.1% of patients were symptomatic for greater than 2 years before diagnosis, and that those aged 36 or less, and those with a history of sleep apnea or obstructive airways disease are at a particularly high risk for being overlooked.

Patients with PH are unable to increase cardiac output during exercise, leading to the initial symptoms of dyspnea on exertion and fatigue. As the disease state progresses the right ventricle undergoes hypertrophy and heart failure develops. Late symptoms include chest pain on exertion, syncope, lower extremity edema, anorexia, and abdominal pain secondary to hepatic congestion.

Bedside cardiac examination may offer clues to clinicians to diagnose PH. Patients with PH may present with a low-normal systolic blood pressure and a loud P2 with a narrow splitting of the second heart sound on auscultation in the early stages. As the right ventricular hypertrophy progresses, jugular venous pressure may be noted with a prominent 'a' wave. Late signs of PH are those of right heart failure and include the presence of a third heart sound, hepatomegaly, peripheral edema, ascites, and pleural effusion.[6,33]

The World Health Organization has developed a functional classification system for patients suffering from PH:

- Class I includes patients without limitations to physical activity
- Class II patients experience slight limitations to physical activity, such as fatigue or dyspnea with normal physical activity

- Class III patients experience marked limitations to physical activity
- Class IV patients are symptomatic at rest and are unable to undergo physical activity

Although there are several different causes that lead to the development of PH, identifying the proper cause is particularly important in guiding the management of the disease. In those with suspected PH, echocardiogram is an appropriate initial screening tool. Characteristic echocardiographic changes in those with PH include enlargement of the right ventricle and atrium, right ventricular hypertrophy, tricuspid regurgitation, or paradoxic motion of the interventricular septum.[34] For those patients in whom there is no evidence of significant left heart disease to explain the PH, other tests should be considered to narrow down the cause.

Findings on chest radiograph may include enlargement of the central pulmonary arteries, right ventricular enlargement as evidenced by encroachment of the retrosternal space, and a prominent right heart border representing right atrial dilation.[6] Electrocardiogram may show evidence of right ventricular hypertrophy. Although these findings may be specific for PAH, they are neither sensitive, nor do they have any indication of disease severity or prognosis.[35] Pulmonary functions tests can be used to identify patients with obstructive versus restrictive disease as possible causes. Additionally, studies have shown a correlation between a decrease in diffusion capacity of carbon monoxide and disease severity.[6,36] Because obstructive sleep apnea has been identified as a cause of PH, polysomnography could be considered in those who are overweight and have a history of snoring. V/Q scan is a highly sensitive and highly specific test that is used for the evaluation of chronic thromboembolic PH. If positive, pulmonary angiography is required to confirm and define the severity of disease. If neither left heart disease nor lung disease are determined to be the cause of PH, blood tests, such as human immunodeficiency infection assay, liver function tests, rheumatoid factor, and antinuclear antibody should be considered.

Definitive diagnosis of PH requires right heart catheterization and is defined as a mean PAP greater than 25 mm Hg at rest. Further classification into the appropriate category often requires additional studies. Diagnosis of PAH requires PAP greater than 25 mm Hg, a mean pulmonary capillary wedge pressure less than 15 mm Hg, and a PVR of greater than 3 Woods units. Additionally, chronic lung disease, venous thromboembolic disease, and other systemic disorders should be ruled out by the clinician. Criteria for diagnosis of category 2, or PH caused by left heart disease, requires PAP greater than or equal to 25 mm Hg, a mean pulmonary capillary wedge pressure greater than or equal to 15 mm Hg, and normal or reduced cardiac output. Diagnosis of category 3 PH requires a PAP greater than or equal to 25 mm Hg in addition to evidence of severe lung disease. PH caused by chronic thromboembolic pulmonary hypertension is defined by elevated PAP on right heart catheterization with evidence of chronic thromboembolisms on V/Q scan in the absence of other identifiable causes. All others with PH who do not clearly fit may fall under category 5.

VASODILATORS

Although early therapy for some with PH should be directed at the underlying disorder, such as management of left heart disease or chronic hypoxemia, patients with more severe PH or those with PAH require more advanced vasodilator-directed therapy. Current recommendations suggest advanced therapy for those with World Health Organization functional class II, III, and IV PH[37] and for many others with PAH. Advanced therapy is primarily directed at three signaling pathways that are directly related to pulmonary vascular regulation: (1) endothelin, (2) NO, and (3) prostacyclin.

TYPES OF VASODILATORS

Calcium Channel Blockers

Calcium channel blockers have long been the standard of therapy for hypertension and PH. Calcium channel blockers cause a vasodilation of the peripheral vasculature by intimal smooth muscle relaxation reducing cardiac afterload and myocardial oxygen demand. They also exert vasodilatory effects on the coronary arteries, thereby increasing blood flow and increasing oxygen delivery to the heart.[38] Specifically in vascular smooth muscle, calcium channel blockers act on the L-type voltage-gated Ca2+ receptors blocking calcium influx and the subsequent release of calcium stores during membrane depolarization resulting in vasodilation.[39] There are three classes of calcium channel blockers: (1) dihydropyridines, which include nifedipine and nicardipine; (2) phenylalkylamines including verapamil; and (3) benzothiazepines, which includes diltiazem. The dihydropyridenes work on the peripheral vascular system causing the vasodilatory effects on vascular smooth muscle, whereas the nondyhydropyridenes have a direct effect on the cardiac contractility, conductivity, and inotropy. Side effects of nifedipine, for example, include hypotension and reflex tachycardia caused by its potency on systemic vascular resistance, whereas verapamil and diltiazem have greater effect on the AV node and thus must be used with caution in those with ventricular dysfunction. Magnesium is also considered a calcium channel blocker and an indirect vasodilator through its stimulation of prostacyclin and NO.[39]

Inhaled Nitric Oxide

Inhaled NO is a potent treatment of reversible PH.[38] The role of inhaled NO was first described in treatment of acute respiratory distress syndrome in PAP and improving V/Q mismatch without significant effect on systemic vascular resistance.[40] Inhaled NO vasodilatory effect in the pulmonary vasculature is mediated through the activation of guanylyl cyclase, which increases cyclic GMP production in the vascular smooth muscle.[39] Cyclic GMP phosphorylates proteins involved in the control of calcium release and smooth muscle contraction. This leads to the activation of protein kinase G and myosin light chain phosphatase, which causes smooth muscle relaxation. NO is an endogenous compound and is an active metabolite in nitrovasodilators, such as sodium nitroprusside and nitroglycerin. It is also important for mediation of vascular tone.[38] Inhaled NO selectively vasodilates the pulmonary vasculature with little systemic effect because of its rapid breakdown in the bloodstream.[41] The main side effects include rebound hypoxemia, PH if abruptly discontinued, and inhibition of platelets.

Prostacyclin

Prostacyclins are vasodilators that affect PVR through smooth muscle prostinoid receptors resulting in cAMP, activation of pKa, and smooth muscle inhibition. As with other vasodilators mentioned, the primary side effect is systemic hypotension from decreased systemic vascular resistance. Prostacyclin stimulates the release of NO by endothelial cells.[39] There are currently three Food and Drug Administration–approved medications for the treatment of PH: (1) intravenous epoprostenol; (2) inhaled iloprost; and (3) treprostinil, which comes in tablet, subcutaneous, and inhaled preparations.[41]

Endothelin Blockers

Endothelin is associated with heart damage, renal failure, and cerebral vasospasm after subarachnoid hemorrhage. Although there have been multiple attempts to isolate these pathways in those disease processes, none were more successful than in mitigating PH.[42] Endothelin receptor antagonists act on endothelin 1 receptors (ETA and ETB), which are smooth muscle vasoconstrictors. Endothelin 1 receptor activation subsequently activates phospholipase C. ETA activation results in vasoconstriction and neoproliferation, whereas ETB activation results in vasodilation through the release of NO.[42] There are selective ETA blockers and general ETA and ETB blockers.[42] Blocking these receptors can lower blood pressure. There are currently three Food and Drug Administration–approved endothelin blockers: (1) bosentan, (2) ambrisentan, and (3) macitentan.[42]

Diuretics

Diuretics are used to treat congestive heart failure, hypertension, and PH. Diuretics treat hypertension by indirectly decreasing intravascular volume and then directly causing vasodilation of the peripheral arterial system.[39] There are three main classes of diuretics: (1) thiazide diuretics; (2) loop diuretics; and (3) potassium-sparing diuretics, which affect different parts of the nephron. For PH diuretics can decrease effusion, namely pleural and pericardial effusions and improving left heart diastolic function. When administered intravenously, the loop diuretics can reduce the fluid order states of heart failure, cirrhosis, nephrotic syndrome, and PH.[38] Diuretics can also be used to decrease the preload, which is beneficial in the pathophysiology of PH due to right-sided heart failure.[43]

Oxygen

Oxygen as a therapy is beneficial in PH because of its benefits of decreasing pulmonary vasoconstriction in a hypoxic state.[38] Through these effects, disease progression is limited and outcomes are improved.[43] In neonates who develop PH through hypoxic respiratory failure, oxygen treatment has been a mainstay.[44] Initially in the 1990s, 100% fraction of inspired oxygen was used but it was noted that neonatal mortality was decreased by 30% when 21% fraction of inspired oxygen, or room air, was used on term babies. Although data are controversial, generally, the same was noted on babies born before 32 weeks. It is hard to define guidelines of O_2 resuscitation, but generally 21% to 30% is used.[44]

Exercise

Typically exercise has not been recommended in the treatment of PH up until recently.[45] More and more studies have showed that exercise can potentially increase the quality of life in those suffering from PH. The changes seen in exercise therapy included improvement in peak oxygen consumption, change in skeletal muscle fiber, improvement in cardiac function, and improvement in hemodynamics. Recommendations for exercise are limited to those who are clinically stable in their disease process and are on optimal pharmacologic management. Regarding how much to exercise, the studies were more exercise intensive than what the general population may be able to accomplish. Benefits were seen exercising 5 days a week for 2 hours a day, but there may be benefits to exercising a couple of times a week for up to 1 hour, which may be more realistic to the stable PH population. The exercise routine may include strength training, aerobic training, and respiratory muscle training, which may all benefit those with PH.

Pregnancy

Pregnancy is a high risk for women of child-bearing age who have PH with significant morbidity and mortality.[46] Guidelines for women with PH are to avoid pregnancy and early termination, although there have been some advances in the treatment of PH recently. Hemodynamically speaking, pregnancy results in plasma volume expansion and an increase in stroke volume, and subsequent increase in cardiac output with reduction in PVR. In normal physiology, the pulmonary vasculature is compliant and can adapt to this change. However, in those with PH, that compliance is decreased and the pulmonary vasculature cannot respond to the decreased resistance, causing an increase in pulmonary pressures resulting in right ventricular failure. If contraception and termination of the pregnancy are not an option for those with PH, the treatment approach should involve multiple providers and specialists and medical management to include calcium channel blockers, PDE-5 inhibitors, and prostacyclins. In addition, delivery should be at 34 weeks and combination spinal-epidural anesthesia should be used with avoidance of large physiologic shifts in blood pressure, heart rate, and volume status.

ANESTHETIC CONSIDERATIONS IN PULMONARY HYPERTENSION

Preoperative

In the preoperative period, patients should continue any treatments for chronic PH. Those medications should be continued before and after any surgery.[43] In newly diagnosed hypertension, sildenafil and 1-arginine are possible treatments preoperatively. Inhaled NO and prostacylcins may confer some benefit if needed and should be available. Propofol, opiates, and neuromuscular blockers can all be used, whereas etomidate and ketamine should be closely monitored because of their suppression of the vasodilating effects in the pulmonary system. Considerations regarding the surgery being performed should be discussed ahead of time. The insufflation in laparoscopic surgery can cause some drastic physiologic changes that are usually tolerated in the general population. In those with PH, insufflation can cause acidosis through P_{CO_2} increase, P_{O_2} decrease, and an increase in the PVR. Certain studies should be obtained before any surgery or procedure. Those studies include complete blood count to check hemoglobin and hematocrit, comprehensive metabolic panel for renal and liver function, electrocardiogram, blood-urea-nitrogen, chest radiograph, and echocardiogram.[1]

Perioperative

There is an increased risk of patients with PH having right-sided heart failure and that risk can increase under anesthesia.[43] This happens in part to the rapid fluctuations and changes in the hemodynamic status of any given patient under anesthesia. Specifically, right ventricular afterload is increased, preload is decreased, hypoxia, and decreased blood pressure can exacerbate the disease process. It is critical to closely monitor patients during induction. The transition from spontaneous breathing to positive pressure and the addition of positive end-expiratory pressure can increase right ventricular afterload. Diuretics are useful intraoperatively, especially if a patient shows signs of hypervolemia, pleural, and/or pericardial effusions. They must be used with caution because of the reduction in preload associated with diuretic use. Intraoperative monitoring is crucial for patients with PH. This includes placement of a central venous catheter with or without Swan-Ganz for monitoring central venous pressure and PAP and placement of an arterial line for monitoring systemic pressures. In addition transesophageal echocardiography is beneficial for the visual interpretation of right ventricular function and volume status.[47] These modalities allow the anesthesiologist to closely monitor subtle changes in the hemodynamic status of the patient. Vasopressors may be used to treat hypotension, whereas vasodilators may be used to treat severe PH. Fluid status and ventilator settings should be maximized to prevent reductions in venous return to the right heart. The typical inhalational anesthetics can markedly decrease the right ventricular contractility. Studies indicate that isoflurane and desflurane increase right ventricular afterload, whereas sevoflurane does seem to affect modification of PVR. One of the inherent risks in anyone with PH during surgery is acute right ventricular failure. The treatment strategy is based on decreasing PVR while stabilizing hemodynamic status with drugs that directly target the pulmonary vasculature. In this regard, inhaled NO and prostacyclins, and the PDE-3 inhibitor milrinone, have all demonstrated clinical benefits.

Postoperative

The same risks are present postoperatively as they are preoperatively. Fluid balance, hemodynamic status, and oxygenation should all be watched closely for any changes. Patients with PH are at an increased risk of worsening disease, pulmonary embolism, cardiac dysfunction, and volume changes and thus should be monitored in the intensive care unit.[47] A multilevel approach should be used for pain management including regional blocks for minimal opioid requirement. The main cause of death postoperatively in someone with PH is respiratory failure and right heart failure leading to arrhythmias. Fluid status must be closely monitored because that can have a tragic effect on precipitating right ventricular failure if preload is increased because of volume overload.

SUMMARY

Patients with PH are at increased risk for morbidity and mortality, including intraoperatively and postoperatively. Appreciation by the clinical anesthesiologist of the pathophysiology of PH is warranted. Careful and meticulous strategy using appropriate anesthetic medications, pulmonary vasodilator and inotropic agents, and careful fluid management all can increase the likelihood of the best possible outcome in this challenging patient population.

REFERENCES

1. Pilkington SA, Taboada D, Martinez G. Pulmonary hypertension and its management in patients undergoing non-cardiac surgery. Anaesthesia 2015;70(1):56–70.
2. Ramakrishna G, Sprung J, Ravi BS, et al. Impact of pulmonary hypertension on the outcomes of noncardiac surgery: predictors of perioperative morbidity and mortality. J Am Coll Cardiol 2005;45(10):1691–9.
3. George MG, Schieb LJ, Ayala C, et al. Pulmonary hypertension surveillance: United States, 2001 to 2010. Chest 2014;146(2):476–95.
4. Ling Y, Johnson MK, Kiely DG, et al. Changing demographics, epidemiology, and survival of incident pulmonary arterial hypertension: results from the pulmonary hypertension registry of the United Kingdom and Ireland. Am J Respir Crit Care Med 2012;186(8):790–6.
5. Humbert M, Sitbon O, Chaouat A, et al. Pulmonary arterial hypertension in France: results from a national registry. Am J Respir Crit Care Med 2006; 173(9):1023–30.
6. Rich JD, Rich S. Clinical diagnosis of pulmonary hypertension. Circulation 2014; 130(20):1820–30.
7. Tolliver BK, McRae-Clark AL, Saladin M, et al. Determinants of cue-elicited craving and physiologic reactivity in methamphetamine-dependent subjects in the laboratory. Am J Drug Alcohol Abuse 2010;36(2):106–13.

8. Hoeper MM, Huscher D, Ghofrani HA, et al. Elderly patients diagnosed with idiopathic pulmonary arterial hypertension: results from the COMPERA registry. Int J Cardiol 2013;168(2):871–80.
9. Galiè N, Manes A, Negro L, et al. A meta-analysis of randomized controlled trials in pulmonary arterial hypertension. Eur Heart J 2009;30(4):394–403.
10. Lajoie AC. Combination therapy versus monotherapy for pulmonary arterial hypertension: a meta-analysis. Lancet Respir. Med 2016;4(4):291–305.
11. Thenappan T, Shah SJ, Rich S, et al. A USA-based registry for pulmonary arterial hypertension: 1982-2006. Eur Respir J 2007;30(6):1103–10.
12. Aaronson PI, Robertson TP, Knock GA, et al. Hypoxic pulmonary vasoconstriction: mechanisms and controversies. J Physiol 2006;570(Pt 1):53–8.
13. Gomazkov OA. The molecular and physiological aspects of endothelial dysfunction. The role of endogenous chemical regulators. Usp Fiziol Nauk 2000;31(4): 48–62 [in Russian].
14. Sandoo A, van Zanten JJ, Metsios GS, et al. The endothelium and its role in regulating vascular tone. Open Cardiovasc Med J 2010;4:302–12.
15. Kubota E, Hamasaki Y, Sata T, et al. Autonomic innervation of pulmonary artery: evidence for a nonadrenergic noncholinergic inhibitory system. Exp Lung Res 1988;14(3):349–58.
16. Benigni A, Cassis P, Remuzzi G. Angiotensin II revisited: new roles in inflammation, immunology and aging. EMBO Mol Med 2010;2(7):247–57.
17. Trask AJ, Ferrario CM. Angiotensin-(1-7): pharmacology and new perspectives in cardiovascular treatments. Cardiovasc Drug Rev 2007;25(2):162–74.
18. Salehi A. Pulmonary hypertension: a review of pathophysiology and anesthetic management. Am J Ther 2012;19(5):377–83.
19. Rudolph AM, Yuan S. Response of the pulmonary vasculature to hypoxia and H+ ion concentration changes. J Clin Invest 1966;45(3):399–411.
20. Subramaniam K, Yared J-P. Management of pulmonary hypertension in the operating room. Semin Cardiothorac Vasc Anesth 2007;11(2):119–36.
21. Zamanian RT, Haddad F, Doyle RL, et al. Management strategies for patients with pulmonary hypertension in the intensive care unit. Crit Care Med 2007;35(9): 2037–50.
22. Fischer LG, Van Aken H, Bürkle H. Management of pulmonary hypertension: physiological and pharmacological considerations for anesthesiologists. Anesth Analg 2003;96(6):1603–16.
23. Kregenow DA, Swenson ER. The lung and carbon dioxide: implications for permissive and therapeutic hypercapnia. Eur Respir J 2002;20(1):1301–8.
24. Hervé P, Launay JM, Scrobohaci ML, et al. Increased plasma serotonin in primary pulmonary hypertension. Am J Med 1995;99(3):249–54.
25. Heath D, Smith P, Gosney J, et al. The pathology of the early and late stages of primary pulmonary hypertension. Br Heart J 1987;58(3):204–13.
26. Liu F, Ventura F, Doody J, et al. Human type II receptor for bone morphogenic proteins (BMPs): extension of the two-kinase receptor model to the BMPs. Mol Cell Biol 1995;15(7):3479–86.
27. Derynck R, Zhang YE. Smad-dependent and Smad-independent pathways in TGF-beta family signalling. Nature 2003;425(6958):577–84.
28. MacLean MR. Endothelin-1 and serotonin: mediators of primary and secondary pulmonary hypertension? J Lab Clin Med 1999;134(2):105–14.
29. Tuder RM, Marecki JC, Richter A, et al. Pathology of pulmonary hypertension. Clin Chest Med 2007;28(1):23–42, vii.

30. Weiss F. Advances in animal models of relapse for addiction research. Boca Raton (FL): CRC Press/Taylor & Francis; 2010.
31. Welsh CH, Hassell KL, Badesch DB, et al. Coagulation and fibrinolytic profiles in patients with severe pulmonary hypertension. Chest 1996;110(3):710–7.
32. Brown LM, Chen H, Halpern S, et al. Delay in recognition of pulmonary arterial hypertension: factors identified from the REVEAL Registry. Chest 2011;140(1): 19–26.
33. Blaise G, Langleben D, Hubert B. Pulmonary arterial hypertension: pathophysiology and anesthetic approach. Anesthesiology 2003;99(6):1415–32.
34. Zee-Cheng CS, Gibbs HR. Paradoxical ventricular septal motion with right ventricular dilatation as a manifestation of pure pressure overload due to pulmonary veno-occlusive disease. Clin Cardiol 1985;8(11):603–6.
35. Ahearn GS, Tapson VF, Rebeiz A, et al. Electrocardiography to define clinical status in primary pulmonary hypertension and pulmonary arterial hypertension secondary to collagen vascular disease. Chest 2002;122(2):524–7.
36. Meyer FJ, Ewert R, Hoeper MM, et al, German PPH Study Group. Peripheral airway obstruction in primary pulmonary hypertension. Thorax 2002;57(6):473–6.
37. Galiè N, Corris PA, Frost A, et al. Updated treatment algorithm of pulmonary arterial hypertension. J Am Coll Cardiol 2013;62(25 Suppl):D60–72.
38. Butterworth JF, Mackey DC, Wasnick JD, et al. Morgan & Mikhail's Clinical Anesthesiology. New York: McGraw-Hill; 2013.
39. Sear JW. Chapter 23-antihypertensive drugs and vasodilators. In: HCH, Egan TD, editors. Pharmacology and physiology for anesthesia. Philadelphia: Elsevier Saunders; 2013. p. 405–25.
40. Rossaint R, Falke KJ, López F, et al. Inhaled nitric oxide for the adult respiratory distress syndrome. N Engl J Med 1993;328(6):399–405.
41. Cosa N, Costa E. Inhaled pulmonary vasodilators for persistent pulmonary hypertension of the newborn: safety issues relating to drug administration and delivery devices. Med Devices (Auckl) 2016;9:45–51.
42. Kuntz M, Leiva-Juarez MM, Luthra S. Systematic review of randomized controlled trials of endothelin receptor antagonists for pulmonary arterial hypertension. Lung 2016;194(5):723–32.
43. Hines RL, Marschall KE. Chapter 5. Systemic and pulmonary arterial hypertension. In: Hines RL, Marschall KE, editors. Stoelting's anesthesia and co-existing disease. 2012. p. 104–19.
44. Lakshminrusimha S, Saugstad OD. The fetal circulation, pathophysiology of hypoxemic respiratory failure and pulmonary hypertension in neonates, and the role of oxygen therapy. J Perinatol 2016;36(Suppl 2):S3–11.
45. Chia KS, Wong PK, Faux S, et al. The benefit of exercise training in pulmonary hypertension: a clinical review. Intern Med J 2016. [Epub ahead of print].
46. Svetlichnaya J, Janmohammed M, De Marco T. Special situations in pulmonary hypertension: pregnancy and right ventricular failure. Cardiol Clin 2016;34(3): 473–87.
47. Fox DL, Stream AR, Bull T. Perioperative management of the patient with pulmonary hypertension. Semin Cardiothorac Vasc Anesth 2014;18(4):310–8.

Alpha-2 Agonists

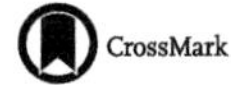

Viet Nguyen, MD[a], Dawn Tiemann, MD[a], Edward Park, MD[b], Ali Salehi, MD[b,*]

KEYWORDS

- Clonidine • Dexmedetomidine • Alpha-2 adrenoreceptors • Pons • Locus coeruleus
- Medullospinal tracts • Dorsal horn • Premedication

KEY POINTS

- Clonidine and dexmedetomidine are alpha-1 and alpha-2 receptor agonists. Dexmedetomidine is a highly selective alpha-2 receptor agonist with an affinity 8 times greater than clonidine for the alpha-2 receptor.
- Their sedative effect is modulated by affecting the pontine locus coeruleus, which is the center for the sympathetic outflow to the forebrain.
- They affect the vasomotor centers of the rostral ventrolateral medulla, which leads to vasodilatation and bradycardia. This action can be associated with an increase in the activity in the parasympathetic neurons.
- Their application is increasing in clinical anesthesia practice. They are used for premedication, sedation, analgesia, and as adjuvants to general and regional anesthesia.
- They have a good safety profile with few side effects, which include hypotension, bradycardia, and sometimes airway obstruction associated with dexmedetomidine.

The 2 major drugs in this category of alpha-2 agonists that are commonly used in anesthesia practice are clonidine and dexmedetomidine, and these are discussed in this article.

CLONIDINE

Introduction

Clonidine, an alpha-2 agonist, is most widely known and used as an antihypertensive agent. Although most of the focus on clonidine is on its ability to reduce blood pressure, it also has sedative and analgesic effects that are of particular interest in anesthesiology.[1–3] Because of its sedative effects, clonidine has long been used as an adjuvant to other anesthetic agents. It also has been used as a premedication to

[a] Department of Anesthesiology, LSUHSC-NO, 1542 Tulane Avenue, Room 659, New Orleans, LA 70112, USA; [b] Department of Anesthesiology and Perioperative Medicine, Ronald Regan UCLA Medical Center, 757 Westwood Plaza, Suite 3325, Los Angeles, CA 90095-7403, USA
* Corresponding author.
E-mail address: asalehi@mednet.ucla.edu

Anesthesiology Clin 35 (2017) 233–245
http://dx.doi.org/10.1016/j.anclin.2017.01.009
anesthesiology.theclinics.com
1932-2275/17/

sedate children before surgery as well as a sedative agent in the pediatric intensive care unit (ICU).[4] Its analgesic effects have also been appreciated as adjuvant to regional and general anesthesia in both the pediatric and adult populations. Because of the effects of clonidine on the cardiovascular system it can be beneficially used in operative cases in which controlled hypotension is desired.[2] Although there are benefits of clonidine usage in anesthesia, care and vigilance must be maintained during the operative process and throughout the perioperative period because adverse effects do occur. Abrupt withdrawal of clonidine can lead to extreme rebound hypertension resulting in hypertensive crisis perioperatively. Clonidine has been shown to decrease the minimum alveolar concentration (MAC) of sevoflurane, so adjustments must be made accordingly.[1,5]

Mechanism of Action

Clonidine produces its effects by stimulating alpha-2 adrenergic receptors in the brainstem. This stimulation in turn activates inhibitory neurons, resulting in decreased central nervous system sympathetic outflow. Decreased outflow manifests in decreased peripheral vascular resistance, decreased renal vascular resistance, and decreases in heart rate and blood pressure. Stimulation of different subtypes of the alpha-2-adrenoreceptor produces particular effects.[1,6]

There are 3 subtypes of adrenergic receptors: alpha-2a, alpha-2b, and alpha-2c.[1]

- Sedation, analgesia, and sympatholysis are produced by stimulating alpha-2a receptors.
- Stimulation of the alpha-2b receptor subtype results in vasoconstriction and trigger antishivering mechanisms.
- Activation of alpha-2c receptors produces the startle response, which in humans results in withdrawal from stimuli, contraction of the extremity muscles, blinking, and variation in blood pressure and breathing patterns.
- Clonidine acts on centrally located alpha-2 receptors, with varying stimulation on all alpha-2 subtypes creating different manifestations.

Pontine locus coeruleus is one of the centrally located areas of alpha-2 receptors that clonidine affects. This area is chiefly responsible for sympathetic nervous system innervations of the forebrain, which is responsible for vigilance. Sedative effects of clonidine result from stimulation of alpha-2 receptors in this area.[1]

Clonidine also activates receptors in the medullary motor center. Clonidine's action in this centrally located area results in a multitude of effects:

- Decreased sympathetic nervous system outflow from the medulla to peripheral nerves, which results in peripheral vasodilatation and a decrease in blood pressure, heart rate, and cardiac output.
- Modification of the potassium channels by clonidine in the neurons in the central nervous system, which causes hyperpolarization of their cell membranes. It has been postulated that this is the mechanism for the recognized decrease in anesthetic requirements attributed to clonidine.

In addition, there are alpha-2 adrenoreceptors located both peripherally and centrally in the neuraxium. Application of clonidine in these areas leads to the inhibition of the release of spinal substance P and nociceptive neuron transmission after stimulation by noxious stimuli. Clonidine's analgesic effects are caused by decreasing pain by stimulating the alpha-2 adrenoreceptors in this area; specifically, at the presynaptic and postsynaptic receptors in the spinal cord, thereby preventing pain signal transmission to the brain.[7–9]

Pharmacokinetics and Pharmacodynamics

Clonidine can be administered intravenously, orally, neuraxially, and transdermally. Clonidine is highly lipid soluble with a volume of distribution of 2.9 L/kg in adults and readily distributes to extravascular sites. When administered in the epidural space, clonidine distributes into the plasma through the epidural veins reaching clinically significant concentrations. Clonidine is rapidly absorbed after oral administration, achieving peak plasma concentration within 60 to 90 minutes. Antihypertensive effects orally are seen within 0.5 to 1 hour. When administered transdermally, full antihypertensive effects of clonidine are reached within 48 to 72 hours. Bioavailability of clonidine is about 75% to 95% with 20% to 40% of the drug being protein bound. Elimination is via hepatic metabolism to inactive metabolites, which are excreted in the urine 40% to 60% unchanged.

Clearance of clonidine is age dependent and differs between neonates and adults. Neonatal clearance is one-third that of adults until age 1 year. At age 1 year, clonidine clearance reaches 82% of an adult's clearance. Neonatal elimination half-life is 44 to 72 hours, in children it is 8 to 12 hours, and in adults it is 12 to 16 hours. Cerebrospinal fluid elimination half-life is 1.3 hours and transdermal half-life elimination is approximately 20 hours after removal of the patch.[5,6,9]

Anesthetic Considerations

Central nervous system

Clonidine decreases both the sympathetic outflow and A delta and C fiber–mediated somatosympathetic reflexes. The result is sedation, analgesia, and reduction in requirement for other anesthetic agents. Cerebral blood flow, cerebral metabolic rate of oxygen, and intraocular pressure also decrease as a result.

Cardiovascular system

Manifestations result from the clonidine-mediated central decrease in sympathetic activity and in turn an increase in vagal tone, which leads to an overall decrease in heart rate and blood pressure. Systemic vascular resistance is also decreased, whereas there is no effect on cardiac contractility, and cardiac output is well maintained.[9,10]

Respiratory system

There is very little respiratory depression. There is no change in respiratory rate, $Paco_2$, or oxygen saturation pressure (Spo_2) on administration.[9]

Renovascular system

Clonidine decreases renovascular resistance and promotes diuresis. Plasma catecholamine concentrations and plasma renin activity are decreased.

Endocrine

Blood glucose levels have been shown to increase because of inhibition of insulin release secondary to the decrease in sympathetic activity.

Clonidine use can be complicated by coadministration of other medications. Acute clonidine or dexmedetomidine (alpha-2 agonist) administration decreases anesthetic requirements by 40% to 60% and chronic administration decreases requirements by 10% to 20%. Tricyclic antidepressant, phenothiazines, and butyrophenones also interfere with the action of clonidine. In addition, clonidine potentiates opiate-induced respiratory depression. Care must be taken to adjust coadministered medications appropriately so as to avoid underdosing/overdosing and the potentiation of other undesired effects.[1,5,9]

Anesthetic Applications

Because of the unique mechanism of action of clonidine, it possesses many properties that can be taken advantage of in an anesthetic setting.

Sedation

The sedation caused by alpha-2 agonists like clonidine differs from the sedation caused by drugs, such as midazolam, that act on gamma-aminobutyric acid (GABA) receptors. Clonidine asserts effects mainly by decreasing the sympathetic nervous system activity and the level of consciousness. This process results in sedation without the risk of respiratory depression and patients can easily be aroused back to full consciousness quickly. No negative effects on cognition, memory, and behavior occur. There is no clouding of consciousness, paradoxic agitation, or tolerance/ dependence anticipated, thus clonidine is regularly considered by some clinicians as a sedative option for the outpatient population.[1,5]

Anesthesia and analgesia adjuvant

Clonidine has been recommended to be used as an anesthetic adjuvant with local anesthetics for regional techniques. This use is especially important in the children because of their narrow therapeutic window and increased incidence of toxicity with regional techniques.[11] The incidence of side effects is lower with clonidine as an adjuvant as opposed to morphine. With clonidine as an adjuvant to regional anesthetic techniques, some clinicians have also found lower incidences of postoperative nausea and vomiting (PONV) and urinary retention.[12] Epidural clonidine can also be used to treat chronic pain. Clonidine can be mixed with hydromorphone and delivered by implantable intrathecal pump for long-term use.[2]

Clonidine improves the analgesic effects of antiinflammatory agents and has peripheral (intra-articular, intravenous, regional) antinociceptive effects in combination with local anesthetics, opioids, and ketamine. Therefore, it can be used in conjunction with other nonopioids to decrease the amount of total opioid use.[1]

As stated earlier, clonidine has been shown to decreases MAC requirements for inhalational agents, particularly with the volatile anesthetic sevoflurane. The MAC of sevoflurane with clonidine was found to be lower than MAC with sevoflurane alone. Clinicians can take advantage of this to decrease patient exposure to volatile inhaled anesthetics.[1,5]

Topical applications

Clonidine can be used as a transdermal patch and topical gel. Both of these have been used with good success rates in painful diabetic neuropathy. Surgical site infiltration with bupivacaine-clonidine combination was recently found to be effective in preventing chronic pain following mastectomy.[1]

Premedication

Clonidine has been used to prevent PONV. It has been used orally and in caudal nerve blocks for this purpose. Clonidine has also been used for treatment of postoperative shivering and for sedation in the ICU.[13–15]

The cardiovascular effects of the drug make it acceptable for usage in cases that require controlled hypotension.[1,2,13]

Adverse Effects

Side effects of clonidine administration have been found to include:

- Drowsiness
- Dry mouth

- Bradycardia
- Orthostatic hypotension
- Impotence
- Rebound hypertension

Rebound hypertension often occurs with the sudden withdrawal of clonidine before surgery. This withdrawal leads to severe hypertension, often resulting in a hypertensive crisis. Therefore, it is recommended that clonidine be continued throughout the perioperative period. It is also recommended that blood glucose be monitored with the use of clonidine because levels may increase because of the inhibition of insulin release by clonidine.

Contraindications

As with any anesthetic drug, vigilance is imperative when using clonidine. Clonidine is contraindicated in patients found to have:

- Hypovolemia
- Atrioventricular block
- Prolonged P-R interval
- Spontaneous bradycardia

Summary

Clonidine is the first congener of alpha-2 adrenergic receptor agonist. It is a mixed alpha-1 and alpha-2 adrenoceptor agonist with a predominant alpha-2 action.[1,2] Clonidine is mainly used as an antihypertensive drug in clinical medicine. However, because of the unique mechanism of action of clonidine, it has also been used for drug detoxification, pain relief, and sedation. Because of the sedative and analgesic effects of clonidine, it is gaining popularity in anesthesiology as an alternative and adjuvant to traditional treatments. It can be used to premedicate children and as an adjuvant to regional and general anesthesia in both pediatric and adult populations. Clonidine has found use in the pediatric ICU as a sedative and analgesic with hemodynamic stability.

Clonidine has a well-established role in acute perioperative pain management. It has been used as an adjuvant to other nonopioid and opioid analgesics, thus allowing decreases in cumulative opioid use. Clonidine has also been used successfully as an adjuvant to neuraxial anesthesia, decreasing the risk of overall toxicity and level of local anesthetic. Recently clonidine has found increasing usage in chronic pain conditions, providing an alternative to traditional pain treatment and better patient satisfaction.[2]

In conclusion, although initially thought of as solely an antihypertensive drug, it is clear that, because of its unique actions on the alpha-2 receptor, clonidine has many more beneficial applications. It is desirable as a premedication with sedative but nonrespiratory depressant properties. Clonidine is used as an adjuvant to analgesics acting both centrally or peripherally. Postoperatively, clonidine treats shivering and PONV or, if administered preoperatively, can perhaps prevent both. Clonidine is a versatile drug with strikingly important and safe properties, and is useful throughout the perioperative period.[1,13]

DEXMEDETOMIDINE

Introduction

Dexmedetomidine is a highly selective alpha-2 adrenergic receptor agonist that confers sedative, anxiolytic, analgesic, and sympatholytic properties; importantly, these effects are achieved with little to no observed respiratory depression at clinically relevant doses.[6] It also produces a level of sedation that is characterized by a level of comfort and ease of arousability in patients that allows their participation in continual assessment.

Dexmedetomidine was initially approved by the United States Food and Drug Administration (FDA) in 1999 for the short-term sedation of intubated and mechanically ventilated patients. In 2008, its approved applications were expanded to include sedation during the perioperative period and in procedural settings.[16] Dexmedetomidine is most commonly delivered intravenously but can also be administered as an oral, sublingual, intranasal, and even intramuscular premedication in uncooperative children and adults. It has also been used as an adjunct medication in locoregional techniques given via both peripheral nerve blocks and neuraxial (intrathecal, epidural, and caudal) administration.

Mechanism of Action

Dexmedetomidine displays approximately 8 times greater affinity for the alpha-2 receptor than does the prototypical alpha-2 agonist clonidine, with a reported affinity for the alpha-2 adrenergic receptor that is roughly 1600 times greater than that of the alpha-1 adrenergic receptor.[17] These G-protein transmembrane alpha-2 receptors are distributed throughout the body to presynaptic, postsynaptic, and extrasynaptic sites of activity, but many of the effects of dexmedetomidine are caused by interactions with alpha-2 receptors located within the brain and spinal cord.

Within the central nervous system, alpha-2 receptors are primarily concentrated within the pons and the medulla of the brainstem and are largely responsible for the transmission of sympathetic activity to the peripheral nervous system. Presynaptic alpha-2 agonism by dexmedetomidine in these areas leads to decreased norepinephrine efflux to the autonomic nervous system, whereas postsynaptic alpha-2 receptor stimulation causes hyperpolarization of neuronal membranes. Dexmedetomidine also exerts effects at both spinal and supraspinal sites of action to modulate nociceptive input and transmission and thus provide analgesia, whereas, in the periphery, alpha-2 receptors in vascular smooth muscle help to mediate vasoconstriction with the more abundant alpha-1 receptors.

Pharmacokinetics and Pharmacodynamics

Alpha-2 receptor activation and modulation by dexmedetomidine occur at different levels of the central and peripheral nervous systems:

- Locus coeruleus; the pontine center of norepinephrine synthesis that mediates vigilance and arousal, and leads to sedation and hypnosis.[18] This mechanism of action is unique in that it does not seem to originate through a GABA-mediated pathway, as occurs with other anxiolytic and sedative-hypnotic agents. As such, dexmedetomidine seems to be devoid of clinically significant respiratory side effects, as shown by only a mild increase in arterial $Paco_2$ and a mild decrease in minute ventilation, even at high doses, and often produces profound sedation.[19]
- Descending medullospinal noradrenergic pathways involved in nociceptive transmission that originate in the locus coeruleus can be inhibited through a presynaptic alpha2–mediated negative feedback mechanism that governs norepinephrine release.
- Rostral ventrolateral medulla; the vasomotor center of the brain that controls sympathetically mediated cardiovascular responses. The presynaptic neuronal

pathway inhibition by dexmedetomidine, combined with activation of parasympathetic neurons in the nucleus ambiguous of the medullary reticular formation, leads to the clinically observed side effects of bradycardia and vasodilatory hypotension seen with its use.
- Spinal effects via alpha-2 agonism within the dorsal horn, which decreases the release of excitatory neurotransmitters, such as glutamate and substance P, thereby reducing ascending spinal pathways involved in nociception and contributing to its analgesic efficacy.[20]

Dexmedetomidine is a lipophilic molecule that is highly bound to plasma proteins, with a large volume of distribution, and is rapidly redistributed to peripheral tissues. It has a distribution half-life of about 6 minutes and shows linear pharmacokinetics over a 24-hour period in patients with normal hepatic and renal function. The context-sensitive half-time of dexmedetomidine can range anywhere from 4 minutes after a 10-minute bolus to more than 250 minutes after an 8-hour continuous infusion.[21] It shows an elimination half-life of approximately 2 hours, undergoes hepatic metabolism via both direct glucuronidation and biotransformation by cytochrome P2A6 oxidation, and is excreted primarily in the urine, with a small amount eliminated in the feces.[22]

Anesthetic Considerations

Initially, the FDA approved dexmedetomidine only for short-term sedation, because of concerns of potential rebound hypertension and tachycardia, given its similarity in mechanism of action to clonidine. These concerns, as yet, do not seem to be warranted, because dexmedetomidine has been used for prolonged durations in the ICU setting without any observed cardiovascular sequelae associated with its subsequent discontinuation. Similarly, withdrawal symptoms seem to be lacking in the setting of prolonged duration of use at this time.

Because it is metabolized extensively through hepatic biotransformation, the judicious use of dexmedetomidine may be warranted in patients with liver disease or failure, because its pharmacokinetic profile may be altered in this setting.

Anesthetic Applications

As described earlier, dexmedetomidine produces many physiologic effects that can be used to great effect in the clinical practice of anesthesiology.

Sedation

Dexmedetomidine use leads to an unconscious state resembling what occurs during natural sleep and may involve cortical and thalamic pathways. This sedative state allows a fairly cooperative, seamless transition from an asleep state to one of wakefulness with stimulation that is devoid of the disinhibition commonly observed with benzodiazepines and other GABA agonists.[23] Multiple trials and meta-analyses also suggest that dexmedetomidine use is associated with less delirium and cognitive disturbance, faster weaning from mechanical ventilation, and decreased time to extubation compared with other sedative agents.[24–28] As such, dexmedetomidine seems to be an ideal primary anesthetic agent in the sedation of intubated and mechanically ventilated patients in the ICU.

Anxiolysis and premedication

Dexmedetomidine's anxiolytic affect, along with the ability to administer it via different routes (oral, sublingual, intranasal, and intramuscular), presents it as an ideal premedicating agent, which is especially important in the pediatric patient population, in whom its advantages include:

- Ease of separation anxiety
- Tolerance of obtaining intravenous access and mask induction
- Prevention of emergence delirium

The intranasal application is especially important in the preoperative treatment of uncooperative adult and pediatric patients without intravenous access because of its ease of administration, avoiding the delayed onset often associated with enteral absorption and bypassing the first-pass effect through the liver.[29,30] To reduce nasal irritation it can be used via nebulizer.

Procedural sedation and monitored anesthesia care

Dexmedetomidine use should be strongly considered as a potential primary or adjunct agent in the sedation of patients undergoing both minor surgical and interventional procedures, especially in those populations in whom hypoventilation and its subsequent effects might be poorly tolerated. Dexmedetomidine seems to induce a state of hypercapnic arousal through its mild increase in arterial $Paco_2$ that allows hyperventilation and partial awakening during deeper levels of sedation without leading to significant respiratory depression.[31] Note that, because of dexmedetomidine's slow onset and offset times and the need for deeper levels of sedation in more stimulating procedures, its use should be confined to dedicated anesthesia providers who can administer adjunctive analgesic and sedative agents as indicated, as well as appropriately monitoring for potential side effects. One specific indication for dexmedetomidine-induced sedation is awake fiberoptic intubation. When used either as the sole anesthetic agent or in combination with other sedative/hypnotic agents, it can provide a suitable intubating condition as shown by:

- Reasonable patient comfort and satisfaction
- Lower incidence of recall
- Less reactivity to the procedure (defensive posturing, verbalizing objections)
- Lower incidence of clinically significant airway obstruction or hypoxia (better safety profile)
- Potential side effects (bradycardia, hypotension) easily treated with standard pharmacologic agents
- Blunting of the hemodynamic perturbations (hypertension, tachycardia) associated with airway management and intubation[32–36]

Pediatric sedation

Pediatric patients who require frequent sedation for various imaging studies (MRI, computed tomography, and PET) may require higher doses of propofol because of acquired tolerance or concomitant medication use (antiepileptic or antirejection agents). In this patient population dexmedetomidine can be used as a sole agent via constant infusion at higher doses or in combination with propofol at lower doses.[37–39] The use of both agents can potentially reduce postprocedure recovery time.

Adjuvant to general anesthesia

When administered as a systemic adjuvant medication during intraoperative general anesthesia, dexmedetomidine has been shown to reduce intraoperative and postoperative opioid requirements and pain intensity scores.[7,40] It has also been shown that, by decreasing the MAC of volatile anesthetics and intraoperative opioid requirements, it can decrease the incidence of PONV without affecting anesthesia recovery times.[41]

Dexmedetomidine's hemodynamic effects seem to make it a useful agent in deliberate hypotension techniques. By decreasing circulating catecholamine levels, dexmedetomidine may lead to decreased free radical formation, reduced neuronal sensitization to excitatory neurotransmitters, improved cerebral perfusion, and more favorable matching of cerebral metabolic supply and demand, resulting in neuroprotective effects.[8]

Intraoperative and postoperative analgesia

Dexmedetomidine also possesses potent analgesic efficacy and can be used as a systemic adjunct in balanced anesthetic techniques in the attenuation of acute postoperative pain. This property is supported by evidence that the use of dexmedetomidine with opioids and coadministered via patient controlled analgesia with or without a background basal infusion results in a reduction in both opioid consumption and rescue analgesic usage.[42] It also decreases the incidence of pruritus and PONV with no observable increase in adverse side effects (hypotension, bradycardia, respiratory depression, and hypoxia) in this setting.

Locoregional techniques

Dexmedetomidine can be used as an adjuvant medication in locoregional techniques and has been effectively administered as part of peripheral nerve blocks, intravenous regional analgesia, and central neuraxial anesthesia. Dexmedetomidine has been shown to:

- Hasten block onset
- Prolong block duration
- Reduce pain scores
- Reduce early postoperative opioid consumption either with neuraxial blocks or peripheral nerve blocks[43–46]

Bradycardia was noted with all types of neuraxial routes, peripheral nerve blocks, and transverse abdominis plane block.

Postoperative shivering

Dexmedetomidine use is also suggested in the management of postoperative shivering, although its ability to do so seems to be no greater than standard management modalities like forced air warming blankets and opioids. The disadvantages of dexmedetomidine use in this context are increased cost and potential need for prolonged monitoring and observation, especially in the ambulatory surgery setting.

Emergence delirium/agitation

In patients with a known history of emergence delirium/agitation, dexmedetomidine can be used either as a premedication or intraoperatively as a bolus and/or continuous infusion throughout the case. In patients without a history of emergence agitation it can be administered as a bolus dose toward the end of the procedure and before awakening. Smaller doses can be used in the postanesthesia care unit if it reoccurs or persists.[11,47–49]

Adverse Effects

Airway obstruction

Despite its minimal effects on respiratory drive, dexmedetomidine, as with all sedative agents, can produce a clinically significant airway obstruction, especially if used in concert with other medications. Thus, continued monitoring for respiratory compromise is warranted in patients who are not intubated or mechanically ventilated.

Bradycardia and hypotension

These side effects are both dose dependent and multifactorial, because they are mediated through both central and peripheral mechanisms but are not the result of direct myocardial depression. Dexmedetomidine at lower doses leads to decreased central sympathetic outflow by reducing the release of norepinephrine and causing a functional sympatholysis. In addition, an alpha-2 receptor agonism of the dorsal motor nucleus of the vagal nerve at lower doses can lead to parasympathomimetic outflow and increased cardiac vagal activity. In contrast, the use of dexmedetomidine at higher doses can be associated with a transient hypertension that occurs via direct stimulation of both peripheral alpha-1 receptors as well as alpha-2 receptors in the vascular smooth musculature.[50] This condition is usually accompanied by a reflex bradycardia and subsequent decrease in cardiac output.

Contraindications

Because of the bradycardia that is typically observed with its administration, the use of dexmedetomidine should be avoided in patients with clinically significant heart blocks or concomitant bradyarrhythmias. In addition, given its vasodilatory effects, the use of dexmedetomidine may be avoided in patients with significant cardiac valvular stenotic lesions or in clinical settings characterized by extreme hypovolemia.

Summary

Dexmedetomidine is a highly selective alpha-2 receptor agonist. Since its approval by the FDA for sedation in the ICU its applications have expanded significantly because of its unique mechanism of action, minimal effect on the respiratory drive, and ideal safety profile. Dexmedetomidine can be administered through intranasal, sublingual, intramuscular, intravenous, and neuraxial routes. Its applications include premedication for pediatric and adult patient populations, procedural sedation and monitored anesthesia care, adjuvant for general and regional anesthesia, perioperative pain control, and postoperative delirium. In conclusion, it is imperative to remember that, although dexmedetomidine has little effect on the respiratory drive, it still can cause airway obstruction when used with other anesthetic agents.

REFERENCES

1. Basker S, Singh G, Jacob R. Clonidine in paediatrics – a review. Indian J Anaesth 2009;53:270–80.
2. Eisensach JC, De Kock M, Klimscha W. α2-adrenergic agonists for regional anesthesia: a clinical review of clonidine. Anesthesiology 1996;85:655–74.
3. Naas S, Ozair E. Dexmedetomidine in current anaesthesia practice - a review. J Clin Diagn Res 2014;8(10):GE01–4.
4. Jing Wang G, Belley-Coté E, Burry L, et al. Clonidine for sedation in the critically ill: a systematic review and meta-analysis. Syst Rev 2015;4:154.
5. Barash PG, Cullen BF, Stoelting RK, et al. Autonomic nervous system physiology and pharmacology. Clinical anesthesia. 7th edition. Philadelphia: Lippincott Williams & Wilkins; 2013. p. 362–407.
6. Maze M, Tranquilli W. Alpha-2 adrenoceptor agonists: defining the role in clinical anesthesia. Anesthesiology 1991;74(3):581–605.
7. Blaudszun G, Lysakowski C, Elia N, et al. Effect of perioperative systemic α2 agonists on postoperative morphine consumption and pain intensity: systematic review and meta analysis of randomized controlled trials. Anesthesiology 2012; 116(6):1312–22.

8. Farag E, Argalious M, Sessler D, et al. Use of α2-agonists in neuroanesthesia: an overview. Ochsner J 2011;11(1):57–69.
9. Giovannitti JA Jr, Thoms SM, Crawford JJ. Alpha-2 adrenergic receptor agonists: a review of current clinical applications. Anesth Prog 2015;62(1):31–9.
10. Chalikonda SA. Alpha2-adrenergic agonists and their role in the prevention of perioperative adverse cardiac events. AANA J 2009;77(2):103–8.
11. Pickard A, Davies P, Birnie K, et al. Systematic review and meta-analysis of the effects of intraoperative α_2-adrenergic agonists on postoperative behavior in children. Br J Anaesth 2014;112(6):982–90.
12. Prasad R, Rao RR, Turai A, et al. Effect of epidural clonidine on characteristics of spinal anaesthesia in patients undergoing gynecological surgeries: a clinical study. Indian J Anaesth 2016;60(6):398–402.
13. Lewis SR, Nicholson A, Smith AF, et al. Alpha-2 adrenergic agonists for the prevention of shivering following general anaesthesia. Cochrane Database Syst Rev 2015;(8):CD011107.
14. Sahi S, Singh MR, Katyal S. Comparative efficacy of intravenous dexmedetomidine, clonidine, and tramadol in post anesthesia shivering. J Anaesthesiol Clin Pharmacol 2016;32(2):240–4.
15. Cruickshank M, Henderson L, MacLennan G, et al. Alpha-2 agonists for sedation of mechanically ventilated adults in intensive care units: a systematic review. Health Technol Assess 2016;20(25):v–xx, 1–117.
16. Gerlach AT, Murphy CV, Dasta JF. An updated focused review of dexmedetomidine in adults. Ann Pharmacother 2009;43(12):2064–74.
17. Barash PG, Cullen BF, Stoelting RK, et al. Intravenous anesthesia, clinical anesthesia. 7th edition. Philadelphia: Lippincott Williams & Wilkins; 2013. p. p478–500.
18. Gertler R, Brown HC, Mitchell DH, et al. Dexmedetomidine: a novel sedative-analgesic agent. Proc (Baylor Univ Med Cent) 2001;14(1):13–21.
19. Venn RM, Hell J, Grounds RM. Respiratory effects of dexmedetomidine in the surgical patient requiring intensive care. Crit Care 2000;4(5):302–8.
20. Ishii H, Kohno T, Yamakura T, et al. Action of dexmedetomidine on the substantia gelatinosa neurons of the rat spinal cord. Eur J Neurosci 2008;27(12):3182–90.
21. Kaur M, Singh PM. Current role of dexmedetomidine in clinical anesthesia and intensive care. Anesth Essays Res 2011;5(2):128–33.
22. Burbulys D, Kiai K. Chapter 83: Alpha-adrenergic analgesics, dexmedetomidine. In: Sinatra RS, Jahr JS, Watkins-Pitchford JM, editors. The essence of analgesia and analgesics. New York: Cambridge University Press; 2011. p. 335–8.
23. Velly L, Rey M, Bruder N, et al. Differential dynamic of action on cortical and subcortical structures of anesthetic agents during induction of anesthesia. Anesthesiology 2007;107(2):202–12.
24. Venn RM, Bradshaw CJ, Spencer R, et al. Preliminary UK experience of dexmedetomidine, a novel agent for postoperative sedation in the intensive care unit. Anesthesia 1999;54(12):1136–42.
25. Pandharipande PP, Pun BT, Herr DL, et al. Effect of sedation with dexmedetomidine vs lorazepam on acute brain dysfunction in mechanically ventilated patients. J Am Med Assoc 2007;298(22):2644–53.
26. Shehabi Y, Grant P, Wolfenden H, et al. Prevalence of delirium with dexmedetomidine compared with morphine based therapy after cardiac surgery: a randomized controlled trial (DEXmedetomidine COmpared to Morphine - DEXCOM Study). Anesthesiology 2009;111(5):1075–84.

27. Riker RR, Shehabi Y, Bokesch PM, et al. Dexmedetomidine vs midazolam for sedation of critically ill patients: a randomized trial. J Am Med Assoc 2009; 301(5):489–99.
28. Jakob SM, Ruokonen E, Grounds RM, et al. Dexmedetomidine vs midazolam or propofol for sedation during prolonged mechanical ventilation: two randomized controlled trials. J Am Med Assoc 2012;307(11):1151–60.
29. Sheta SA, Al-Sarheed MA, Abdelhalim AA. Intranasal dexmedetomidine vs midazolam for premedication in children undergoing complete dental rehabilitation: a double-blinded randomized controlled trial. Paediatr Anaesth 2014;24(2):181–9.
30. Surendar MN, Pandey RK, Saksena AK, et al. A comparative evaluation of intranasal dexmedetomidine, midazolam and ketamine for their sedative and analgesic properties: a triple blind randomized study. J Clin Pediatr Dent 2014; 38(3):255–61.
31. Rozet I, Souter M, Domino K, et al. Dexmedetomidine sedation for awake craniotomies. Anesthesiology 2004;101(3A):A375.
32. Bergese SD, Patrick Bender S, McSweeney TD, et al. A comparative study of dexmedetomidine with midazolam and midazolam alone for sedation during elective awake fiberoptic intubation. J Clin Anesth 2010;22(1):35–40.
33. Chu KS, Wang FY, Hsu HT, et al. The effectiveness of dexmedetomidine infusion for sedating oral cancer patients undergoing awake fibreoptic nasal intubation. Eur J Anaesthesiol 2010;27(1):36–40.
34. Tsai CJ, Chu KS, Chen TI, et al. A comparison of the effectiveness of dexmedetomidine versus propofol target-controlled infusion for sedation during fibreoptic nasotracheal intubation. Anaesthesia 2010;65(3):254–9.
35. Cattano D, Lam NC, Ferrario L, et al. Dexmedetomidine versus remifentanil for sedation during awake fiberoptic intubation. Anesthesiol Res Pract 2012;2012: 753107.
36. Hu R, Liu JX, Jiang H. Dexmedetomidine versus remifentanil sedation during awake fiberoptic nasotracheal intubation: a double-blinded randomized controlled trial. J Anesth 2013;27(2):211–7.
37. Mason K, Zgleszewski S, Prescilla R, et al. Hemodynamic effects of dexmedetomidine sedation for CT imaging studies. Paediatr Anaesth 2008;18(5):393–402.
38. Mason K, Zurakowski D, Zgleszewski S, et al. High dose dexmedetomidine as the sole sedative for pediatric MRI. Paediatr Anaesth 2008;18(5):403–11.
39. Mason K, Robinson F, Fontaine P, et al. Dexmedetomidine offers an option for safe and effective sedation for nuclear medicine imaging in children. Radiology 2013;267(3):911–7.
40. Schnabel A, Meyer-Frießem CH, Reichl SU, et al. Is intraoperative dexmedetomidine a new option for postoperative pain treatment? A meta-analysis of randomized controlled trials. Pain 2013;154(7):1140–9.
41. Le Bot A, Michelet D, Hilly J, et al. Efficacy of intraoperative dexmedetomidine compared with placebo for surgery in adults: a meta-analysis of published studies. Minerva Anestesiol 2015;81(10):1105–17.
42. Peng K, Liu H, Wu S, et al. Effects of combining dexmedetomidine and opioids for postoperative intravenous patient-controlled analgesia. Clin J Pain 2015;31(12): 1097–104.
43. Abdallah FW, Brull R. Facilitatory effects of perineural dexmedetomidine on neuraxial and peripheral nerve block: a systematic review and meta-analysis. Br J Anaesth 2013;110(6):915–25.

44. Wu HH, Wang HT, Jin JJ, et al. Does dexmedetomidine as a neuraxial adjuvant facilitate better anesthesia and analgesia? A systematic review and meta-analysis. PLoS One 2014;9(3):e93114.
45. Almarakbi WA, Kaki AM. Addition of dexmedetomidine to bupivacaine in transversus abdominis plane block potentiates post-operative pain relief among abdominal hysterectomy patients: a prospective randomized controlled trial. Saudi J Anaesth 2014;8(2):161–6.
46. Qi X, Li Y, Rahe-Meyer N, et al. Intrathecal dexmedetomidine as adjuvant to ropivacaine in hysteroscopic surgery: a prospective, randomized control study. Int J Clin Pharmacol Ther 2016;54(3):185–92.
47. Ali MA, Abdellatif AA. Prevention of sevoflurane related emergence agitation in children undergoing adenotonsillectomy: a comparison of dexmedetomidine and propofol. Saudi J Anaesth 2013;7(3):296–300.
48. Sun L, Guo R, Sun L. Dexmedetomidine for preventing sevoflurane-related emergence agitation in children: a meta-analysis of randomized controlled trials. Acta Anaesthesiol Scand 2014;58(6):642–50.
49. Hauber JA, Davis PJ, Bendel LP, et al. Dexmedetomidine as a rapid bolus for treatment and prophylactic prevention of emergence agitation in anesthetized children. Anesth Analg 2015;121(5):1308–15.
50. Ebert TJ, Hall JE, Barney JA, et al. The effects of increasing plasma concentrations of dexmedetomidine in humans. Anesthesiology 2000;93(2):382–94.

Perioperative Pharmacologic Considerations in Obesity

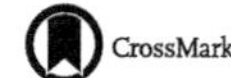

Simon Willis, MD[a], Gregory J. Bordelon, MD[b], Maunak V. Rana, MD[c,*]

KEYWORDS

- Obesity • Anesthesia dosing • Induction • Scalars • Overdose • Morbid obesity

KEY POINTS

- Perioperative physicians must be aware of the physiologic alterations in obese patients because of the increase in incidence of this condition.
- Obese patients have alterations in the pharmacologic responses to induction agents and perioperative physicians should take a tailored approach for anesthetic choices.
- Perioperative physicians should be familiar with common dosing scalars to choose appropriate dosing in patients to avoid both underdosing and overdosing obese patients.

INTRODUCTION

Over the last 3 decades the incidence of morbid obesity has tripled worldwide; at least 5% of the population in the United States is considered morbidly obese.[1] As the incidence of obesity increases, there has been a correlative increase in the incidence of associated comorbidities, including diabetes, cardiopulmonary disease, hypertension, and obstructive sleep apnea. Furthermore, morbid obesity is also associated with important physiologic and anthropometric changes that may alter the pharmacokinetic properties of most anesthetic drugs.[2] As obesity becomes more prevalent in the population, the number of obese patients who require surgical procedures will consequently increase. Associated comorbidities in conjunction with the altered

---

Disclosure: The authors have nothing to disclose.

[a] Department of Physical Medicine and Rehabilitation, MedStar Georgetown University Hospital/National Rehabilitation Hospital, 102 Irving Street Northwest, Washington, DC 20010, USA; [b] Department of Anesthesiology, Louisiana State University Medical Center, 1542 Tulane Avenue, Room 659, New Orleans, LA 70112, USA; [c] Department of Anesthesiology, Advocate Illinois Masonic Medical Center, 836 West Wellington Avenue, Suite 4815, Chicago, IL 60657, USA

* Corresponding author.

E-mail address: maunakr@gmail.com

Anesthesiology Clin 35 (2017) 247–257
http://dx.doi.org/10.1016/j.anclin.2017.01.010
anesthesiology.theclinics.com

pharmacokinetics of obese patients highlight the importance for modern anesthesiologist/periprocedural physicians to understand the increased risks associated with providing anesthesia to this patient population.

EPIDEMIOLOGY

Obesity is a global epidemic that has been increasing in incidence and prevalence. Over the past 30 years, with the evolution of economic prosperity and growth, industrialization, and urbanization, the prevalence of obesity has increased exponentially throughout many countries. Furthermore, a nutritional transition to processed foods and high-calorie diets in combination with an increasingly sedentary lifestyle has driven people into overweight states subsequently caused an increase in associated comorbidities.[3] It is estimated that more than a third of the world's population is affected by obesity.[4] If the current trend of increasing obesity continues, experts predict that 38% of the world's adult population will be overweight by 2030, with another 20% being obese.[5] By 2030 in the United States alone, it is expected that up to 85% of adults will be overweight or obese.[6] In general, the prevalence of obesity is greater in developed countries in patients of a poor socioeconomic status, whereas, in areas of development, the wealthier population is more likely to have a higher portion of obesity.[7]

DEFINITIONS

Contrary to drug dosing in normal-weight patients, dosing scalars in obese patients should reflect and compensate for changes in body composition. Scalars that take into consideration body composition relevant to obese patients include body mass index (BMI), ideal body weight (IBW), lean body weight (LBW), total body weight (TBW), percentage IBW, body surface area (BSA), adjusted body weight, and predicted normal weight.[1] These scalars are metrics that frequently are used to determine dosing of anesthetic agents. On careful consideration, certain scalars are more appropriate and easily adjusted to suit obese patients, with safe and appropriate dosing.

BMI is the most commonly used parameter in the determination and grading of obesity. It takes into consideration both the body weight in kilograms and height in squared meters of the individual, using the formula of body weight (kg)/height (m)^2. Different categories of obesity have been established using various ranges of BMI, with higher BMI correlating with obesity severity. Normal BMI is represented in the range between 20 and 25 kg/m^2. Individuals are classified as overweight with a BMI between 26 and 29 kg/m^2, and obese with a BMI of greater than or equal to 30 kg/m^2. Obesity is further broken down with class I obesity being diagnosed with a BMI of 30 to 34 kg/m^2, class II obesity as 35 to 39 kg/m^2, and class III obesity (formerly known as morbid obesity) as a BMI of greater than 40 kg/m^2. Furthermore, individuals with a BMI of greater than 50 kg/m^2 are considered supermorbidly obese and super-supermorbidly obese with a BMI of greater than 60 kg/m^2.[1]

TBW is a term used in the biological and medical sciences to describe mass or weight, generally measured in kilograms. It represents the weighed body weight of an individual without any added adjustments.

The concept of IBW was developed in both men and women for what was thought to represent a maximally healthy person.[8] It is associated with the maximum life expectancy for people with a particular build, describing a relationship between the idealized weight correlated with height.[1] IBW differs between genders; because it is based on height, it is not a particularly appropriate means of identifying anesthetic doses in obese patients because all patients of the same height receive the same dose.

Furthermore, it does not fully take into account the body composition changes seen in obese individuals. Although there exist many similar equations for calculating IBW, the most commonly used formula for estimating IBW is the Devine formula, represented in men by IBW (in kilograms) = 50 + 2.3 kg per inch more than 5 feet, whereas in women it is IBW (in kilograms) = 45.5 + 2.3 kg per inch more than 5 feet. In calculating IBW for people less than 5 feet (60 inches) tall, the weight per inches factor can merely be subtracted out. A simplified formula has been suggested as well to estimate the IBW, with IBW (in kilograms) = BMI $\times$ height^2 (in meters), with many finding that a BMI of 22 represents the best generic value for both men and women in this formula.[2,9,10] The calculated IBW in morbidly obese patients is less than their LBW; this discrepancy can cause potential underdosing if the administration of a drug is based on LBW. Percentage IBW is represented by the ratio of TBW to IBW, but similarly does not take into consideration body composition variances in obese patients.

LBW is the TBW calculated minus the weight of body fat or fat mass. It includes bones, tendons, ligaments, and body water. In normal men, LBW should be approximately 80% of the TBW, whereas in women it should be represented by 75%. In obese patients, LBW can be estimated by increasing the IBW by close to 20% to 30%. There are several formulas that exist to estimate the lean body mass; however, for morbidly obese patients the most accurate seems to be the Janmahasatian formula. This formula takes into account weight, BMI, and sex to estimate lean body mass. **Table 1** includes this formula, as well as the formulas for all the scalars mentioned earlier.[11]

BSA is the total surface area of the human body. There are multiple equations to approximate the result of the height and weight as the BSA of patients, but the most widely used formula is the Du Bois formula, which has been shown to be equally effective in estimating body fat in obese and nonobese patients.[12,13] The formula is represented by BSA (m^2) = 0.20247 $\times$ height (m)$^{0.725}$ $\times$ weight (kg)$^{0.425}$. Evidence has shown that BSA values are less accurate at height and weight extremes for hemodynamic parameters in which BMI may be a better estimate.[14] In addition, using the BSA scalar is not ideal to calculate drug dose in obese patients because it does not account for differences in body composition.

Adipose tissue distribution is another important factor to consider when evaluating patients for obesity because the objective BMI calculation may not provide an accurate assessment of the patient's tissue composition.[1] There exist 2 types of fat distribution: android and gynecoid.[7] Centrally located android fat is more common in men. It is represented by increased intra-abdominal or visceral fat, which is more metabolically active than peripheral fat. Increased levels of this fat may lead to a greater risk of metabolic derangements. In contrast, gynecoid fat is more peripherally located, being distributed more in the buttocks, hips, and lower extremities.

Table 1
Equations for dosing scalars

BMI (kg/m^2)	Weight (kg)/height (m)^2
TBW (kg)	Measured body weight
IBW (kg)	Men = 50 + (2.3 [height (in) – 60]) Women = 45 + (2.3 [height (in) – 60])
LBW (kg)	Men = (9270 $\times$ TBW)/[6680 + (216 $\times$ BMI)] Women = (9270 $\times$ TBW)/[8780 + (244 $\times$ BMI)]
BSA (m)^2	0.20247 $\times$ height (m)$^{0.725}$ $\times$ weight (kg)$^{0.425}$

PHYSIOLOGIC CHANGES IN OBESITY

Obesity leads to physiologic and anatomic changes that affect the delivery of anesthesia and perioperative analgesia. Many of these changes severely alter the respiratory and cardiovascular systems, which are of utmost concern to the anesthesiology team. Pulmonary changes in obesity with pharmacologic implications include changes in lung volume, respiratory rate, as well as oxygen (O_2) consumption and carbon dioxide (CO_2) production. In obese patients, functional residual capacity (FRC), expiratory reserve volume, as well as total lung capacity (TLC) are all decreased.[15] An exponential relationship between BMI and FRC exists, in which a reduction in FRC may become so pronounced that it approaches residual volume.[16] As a consequence, small airways and alveoli may remain closed during spontaneous ventilation, which can cause a ventilation-perfusion (V/Q) mismatch and right-to-left shunting. This mismatch results in gas exchange abnormalities, with the development of mild hypoxia, which is worse when in the supine position. Similarly, TLC is reduced because the increase in body mass affects the balance of the chest wall forces, including recoil, lung compliance, and the muscle forces involved in the respiratory process through added pressure applied to the chest wall. Obese patients are also at increased risk of developing obstructive sleep apnea (OSA) secondary to increased adiposity, with 50% to 70% of overweight and obese patients having OSA.[17] Moreover, obese patients with OSA have been found to have negative outcomes with anesthesia related to intubation failure, respiratory obstruction soon after extubation, or respiratory arrest after narcotic and sedative medication.[18] As a result, obese patients develop a decreased time to desaturation during apnea, increased O_2 requirements, and hypoventilation with supine spontaneous ventilation.[19–21]

Obese patients also experience physiologic changes to their cardiovascular systems. Cardiac disease is a common problem observed in obese patients, with the American Heart Association (AHA) identifying obesity as an independent risk factor. Obesity causes an increase in circulating blood volume with a decrease in systemic vascular resistance, often resulting in volume overload. Cardiac output increases as well, by 20 to 30 mL per kilogram of excess body fat secondary to a broadened stroke volume. The state of volume overload, with high end-diastolic volumes and increased filling pressure, along with increased cardiac output promotes left ventricular hypertrophy (LVH), in correlation with duration of an obese state. Often the development of LVH leads to left ventricular failure, especially when associated with a comorbid hypertension. Right ventricular failure may develop subsequently in obese patients who have long-standing left ventricular failure or can be seen with hypoxia, hypercapnia (especially common in patients with OSA), and patients with either pulmonary venous or arterial hypertension.

GENERAL DOSING STRATEGIES

Because the pharmacokinetics and pharmacodynamics of anesthetic agents are altered with respect to obese patients, the variability requires careful assessment and evaluation of parameters to observe drug effects, including LBW, fat mass, and extracellular fluid volume. In the past in nonobese patients, TBW was the preferred scalar used to calculate drug dose, despite metabolic processes occurring in lean tissue.[22] Using TBW is a concern in obese patients because the fatty tissue and LBW do not increase in a directly proportional fashion. Instead, as fat tissue increases in proportion to TBW, the ratio of LBW to TBW decreases. This variation affects reliable pharmacokinetic prediction, requiring the use of an alternative scalar when dosing in obesity. Furthermore, cardiac output, another parameter to consider in drug dosage, increases in obese patients compared with nonobese cohorts.[1]

Other factors that affect dosing that need to be taken into consideration when using anesthetics in obesity include volume of distribution (Vd) and drug elimination. Vd is the apparent volume that would be necessary to contain the total amount of an administered drug at the same concentration that it is observed in the blood plasma. Factors that affect Vd include the lipophilicity/hydrophilicity of the drug, lean body mass, fat quantity, cardiac output and circulatory blood volume, total body water, and protein binding of the drug. Increased triglycerides, cholesterol, and fatty acid levels, which are all commonly seen in overweight and obese states, can decrease drug protein binding. One example of this alteration is increased a-1 acid glycoprotein binding of local anesthetics, reducing the amount of free drug in the plasma. Elimination is the process by which the body metabolizes and removes the drug. Phase I and phase II reaction phases determine elimination. Phase I involves redox and hydrolysis reactions and is normal to increased in obese patients. Phase II involves conjugation (glucuronidation), which is increased in obesity. Renal clearance is increased in obesity secondary to increased renal blood flow and glomerular filtration rate. The use of LBW is advocated when considering drug clearance because this process increases linearly with increases in LBW versus nonlinearly for increases in IBW.

ANESTHETIC INDUCTION AGENTS

Despite physiologic changes in obesity compared with nonobese patients, choice of induction agents does not differ. Propofol is the most commonly used agent for the induction and maintenance of anesthesia as well as for the sedation of mechanically ventilated patients. This highly lipophilic agent has a high Vd. It undergoes extensive metabolism in the liver, predominantly through glucuronidation and oxidation, and has a long elimination half-life.[23] A study conducted by Cortinez and colleagues[24] evaluated propofol pharmacokinetics of 19 obese ASA II patients undergoing bariatric surgery to identify the best size descriptor for volumes and clearances in obese patients. The study concluded that an allometric model using TBW was superior to other descriptors for all clearance parameters studied, including linear TBW, free fat mass, LBW, and normal fat mass. No gender effects were found in the results of propofol pharmacokinetics, differing from a prior study.[25] Another study, performed by Dong and colleagues,[26] found that the anesthetic effects of propofol were greatly enhanced in morbidly obese subjects when propofol was dosed using the weight scalar of TBW. In addition, with a dose reduction based on LBW, similar anesthetic effects occurred compared with a nonobese control group of subjects who were dosed using TBW. Furthermore, morbidly obese subjects dosed based on LBW had similar pharmacodynamic effects compared with the control group, indicating that LBW was a better dosing scalar in the morbidly obese cohort.[26]

Adjusted body weight is a modification to the TBW that has been suggested as a way to reliably predict pharmacokinetics in obese patients. One study evaluated 24 patients with BMIs ranging from 35.5 to 61.7 kg/m^2 using a corrected factor to TBW to assess a propofol target–controlled infusion in morbidly obese patients. The corrected weight versus non–weight-adjusted patients were evaluated with drug levels and bispectral index values.[27] Weight adjustment was shown to lead to clinically unacceptable results regarding predictability. Another study, by Albertin and colleagues,[28] found that TBW was corroborated as a more accurate measure of dosing of propofol in obese patients undergoing biliointestinal surgery when coadministered the analgesic remifentanil.

Etomidate is an induction agent used for cardiovascular stability in hemodynamically compromised patients. Etomidate has been recommended to be administered by LBW,[29] but some clinicians have advocated dosing according to IBW in morbidly obese patients.[30]

The pharmacokinetics of ketamine have not been studied in a detailed fashion. This agent is described via a 2-compartment model. The drug is lipophilic with a large Vd. At present, ketamine is recommended to be administered by IBW.[31]

NEUROMUSCULAR BLOCKING AGENTS

Succinylcholine is a depolarizing neuromuscular blocker used to induce muscle relaxation and short-term paralysis to assist in endotracheal intubation. Plasma cholinesterase (PCE) is an enzyme required for the metabolism and breakdown of particular anesthesia-related medications, most notably succinylcholine. In obesity, PCE level increases in direct proportion to body weight, subsequently causing an increased metabolism of succinylcholine. Furthermore, as the extracellular fluid volume is also increased with increasing TBW, the duration of action of succinylcholine is altered. Secondary to these changes, succinylcholine requires an increased absolute dose with a reduced dose per unit body weight during administration.

Vecuronium is another nondepolarizing skeletal muscle relaxant and neuromuscular blocker used to facilitate endotracheal intubation and provide skeletal muscle relaxation during surgery. It is derived from the same aminosteroid structure as pancuronium, which operates by competing for choline receptors at motor end plates, producing a paralytic effect. Obese patients using TBW-based vecuronium took approximately 60% longer to recover from neuromuscular blocking effects compared with another group of nonobese patients. The same study recommended basing administration on IBW in order to prevent and avoid an overdose in obese patients.[32]

Rocuronium bromide is an aminosteroid nondepolarizing neuromuscular blocker and muscle relaxant that is often used during endotracheal intubation. It is weakly lipophilic, which limits distribution outside the extracellular fluid space. Pühringer and colleagues[33] found that rocuronium had a shorter time of onset and mildly longer duration of action in obese patients compared with a group of normal-weight patients. However, a subsequent study found that pharmacokinetic parameters and spontaneous recovery to 75% of twitch height after rocuronium administration were similar in obese and normal-weight subjects.[34] A study in 2004 assessing 12 morbidly obese women presenting for laparoscopic gastric banding surgery found that rocuronium dosing should be based on IBW because TBW dosing was shown to approximately double the duration of action, averaging 55 minutes.[35] Furthermore, onset time of rocuronium was no different when dosed at 0.6 mg/kg based on IBW, IBW and 20% of excess weight, or IBW and 40% of excess weight.[36]

Cisatracurium is another nondepolarizing neuromuscular blocker used for endotracheal intubation and muscle relaxation, now typically administered in patients with hepatic/renal dysfunction. It has similar pharmacokinetics to atracurium because it is one of its 10 stereoisomers. Unlike atracurium, administration of cisatracurium avoids histamine release. Like atracurium, cisatracurium is eliminated via Hoffman degradation. In a study by Leykin and colleagues,[37] the duration of action of cisatracurium was prolonged when dosed according to TBW in morbidly obese patients compared with a control group of nonobese patients. The same study also found prolonged duration of action between morbidly obese patients versus nonobese control patients when dosing of the agent was based on IBW.[37]

REVERSAL AGENTS

Neostigmine is an anticholinesterase that increases the amount of acetylcholine at both the nicotinic and muscarinic receptors and therefore reverses the effects of competitive nondepolarizing neuromuscular blockers. In one study, obese and nonobese patients who received vecuronium based on TBW were compared. After a standard dose of 0.04 mg/kg of neostigmine there was no significant difference in recovery to a train of 4 ratio of 0.7 in obese versus nonobese patients. However, full recovery to a train of 4 ratio of 0.9 was prolonged in obese patients.[38]

Sugammadex is a reversal agent that acts by binding steroidal nondepolarizing neuromuscular blockers to its lipophilic core. Dosing of sugammadex is based on the number of posttetanic twitches or time from administration. Within 3 minutes of an intubating dose (1.2 mg/kg) of rocuronium, the dose of sugammadex should be 16 mg/kg. If the patient has reached 1 to 2 posttetanic twitches the dose should be 4 mg/kg. If there are 2 posttetanic twitches the dose can be decreased to 2 mg/kg. Dosing recommendations from the manufacturer are based on body weight. However, according to Van Lancker and colleagues,[39] dosing sugammadex based on IBW can reliably reverse morbidly obese patients from rocuronium-induced paralysis. They also suggest that dosing to IBW plus 40% decreases the time to full reversal.[39]

INHALED ANESTHETIC AGENTS

Inhaled anesthetics function by uptake of gas from the alveoli and equilibration with the blood and brain. The solubility of the anesthetic determines the speed of uptake and equilibration. More soluble anesthetics must have a large amount dissolved in blood before equilibrium with the brain and effect are achieved. After equilibrium with blood is achieved, other tissues, including muscle and fat, act as a reservoir for inhaled anesthetics. The amount of uptake is a directly related to solubility and length of exposure. When inhaled anesthetic is discontinued, the tissues continue to offset anesthetic and can delay emergence. The solubility of inhaled anesthetics can be defined for each medium (eg, blood, brain, muscle, fat); however, in general it is referred to by the blood-gas partition coefficient. The higher the partition coefficient, the more soluble the gas.[40] **Table 2** lists the partition coefficients for the anesthetics described earlier.

Isoflurane is the most lipophilic of the commonly used inhaled anesthetics. Conceptually this would mean that obesity leads to increased uptake into the adipose tissue, leading to a delayed emergence from anesthesia. However, at 0.6 MAC in procedures lasting 2 to 4 hours there was no significant difference in the time to emergence between obese and nonobese patients. This finding is theorized to be secondary to decreased fat perfusion and increased time constants for isoflurane to equilibrate with fat, therefore negating the excess adipose tissues effect on uptake.[41]

Desflurane is the least lipophilic volatile anesthetic, with a blood gas coefficient of 0.45 and therefore has the least uptake by adipose tissue. Because of this property,

Table 2
Partition coefficients for volatile anesthetics

Volatile Anesthetic	Blood-Gas Partition Coefficient
Isoflurane	1.46
Sevoflurane	0.65
Desflurane	0.45

time to emergence is decreased compared with isoflurane. However, there was no significant difference in the time to emergence in obese versus nonobese patients.[41]

Sevoflurane is half as soluble as isoflurane, with a blood gas coefficient of 0.65. Like desflurane, time to emergence is decreased compared with isoflurane based on the property of lipophilicity.[42] Compared with desflurane, there was no clinically significant reduction in time to emergence with sevoflurane in obese patients.[43]

ANALGESICS

Fentanyl is the most commonly used opioid analgesic used in anesthesia. Obesity itself leads to no change in elimination despite patients having a higher amount of adipose tissue. For drug administration, there should be no change in dose per unit body weight with dosing based on IBW. Dosing may be decreased /because of concerns of respiratory depression.

Sufentanil is a synthetic derivative of fentanyl that is roughly 10 times more potent. It is highly lipophilic and has an increased Vd in obese patients compared with normal-weight individuals, which correlates with the scale of obesity. Furthermore, the increased Vd subsequently results in an increased elimination half-life in obese patients. The slow elimination in obese patients suggests that infusion or maintenance doses should be reduced.[44]

The pharmacokinetics of remifentanil are not appreciably different in obese and lean patients. Dosing of this agent is based on lean body mass or IBW.[45,46]

SUMMARY

Obesity is an epidemic that has greatly affected the practice of medicine, including that of anesthesia. The pharmacokinetics and pharmacodynamics of commonly used drugs can be affected by the increase in adipose tissue. **Table 3** lists recommendations on weight-based dosing of commonly used anesthetic drugs. These recommendations are based on the information and studies presented earlier; however, clinical judgment on a patient-by-patient basis is recommended when dosing drugs.

Table 3
Recommendations on weight-based dosing of commonly used anesthetic drugs

Propofol	Induction: LBW Infusion: TBW
Etomidate	LBW
Ketamine	IBW
Succinylcholine	TBW
Vecuronium	IBW
Rocuronium	IBW
Cisatracurium	IBW
Neostigmine	TBW
Sugammadex	TBW
Fentanyl	IBW
Sufentanil	TBW
Remifentanil	IBW

REFERENCES

1. Lemmens HJ. Perioperative pharmacology in morbid obesity. Curr Opin Anaesthesiol 2010;23(4):485–91.
2. Carron M, Guzzinati S, Ori C. Simplified estimation of ideal and lean body weights in morbidly obese patients. Br J Anaesth 2012;109(5):829–30.
3. Hruby A, Hu FB. The epidemiology of obesity: a big picture. PharmacoEconomics 2015;33(7):673–89.
4. Stevens GA, Singh GM, Lu Y, et al. National, regional, and global trends in adult overweight and obesity prevalences. Popul Health Metr 2012;10(1):22.
5. Kelly T, Yang W, Chen C-S, et al. Global burden of obesity in 2005 and projections to 2030. Int J Obes 2008;32(9):1431–7.
6. Wang Y, Beydoun MA, Liang L, et al. Will all Americans become overweight or obese? estimating the progression and cost of the US obesity epidemic. Obesity (Silver Spring) 2008;16(10):2323–30.
7. Adams JP, Murphy PG. Obesity in anaesthesia and intensive care. Br J Anaesth 2000;85(1):91–108.
8. Pai MP, Paloucek FP. The origin of the "ideal" body weight equations. Ann Pharmacother 2000;34(9):1066–9.
9. Lemmens HJ, Brodsky JB, Bernstein DP. Estimating ideal body weight - a new formula. Obes Surg 2005;15:1082–3.
10. Matsuzawa Y, Tokunaga K, Kotani K, et al. Simple estimation of ideal body weight from body mass index with the lowest morbidity. Diabetes Res Clin Pract 1990;10:S159–64.
11. Coetzee JF. Dose scaling for the morbidly obese: SASA refresher course texts. Southern African Journal of Anaesthesia and Analgesia 2014;20(1):69–72.
12. Du Bois D, Du Bois EF. A formula to estimate the approximate surface area if height and weight be known. 1916. Nutrition 1989;5(5):303.
13. Verbraecken J, Van de Heyning P, De Backer W, et al. Body surface area in normal-weight, overweight, and obese adults. A comparison study. Metabolism 2006;55(4):515–24.
14. Adler AC, Nathanson BH, Raghunathan K, et al. Misleading indexed hemodynamic parameters: the clinical importance of discordant BMI and BSA at extremes of weight. Crit Care 2012;16(6):1.
15. Jones RL, Nzekwu MU. The effects of body mass index on lung volumes. Chest 2006;130(3):827–33.
16. Salome CM, King GG, Berend N. Physiology of obesity and effects on lung function. J Appl Physiol (1985) 2010;108(1):206–11.
17. Young T, Shahar E, Nieto FJ, et al. Predictors of sleep-disordered breathing in community-dwelling adults: the Sleep Heart Health Study. Arch Intern Med 2002;162(8):893–900.
18. Benumof JL. Obesity, sleep apnea, the airway and anesthesia. Curr Opin Anaesthesiol 2004;17(1):21–30.
19. Kabon B, Nagele A, Reddy D, et al. Obesity decreases perioperative tissue oxygenation. Anesthesiology 2004;100(2):274–80.
20. Jense HG, Dubin SA, Silverstein PI, et al. Effect of obesity on safe duration of apnea in anesthetized humans. Anesth Analg 1991;72(1):89–93.
21. Lee MY, Lin CC, Shen SY, et al. Work of breathing in eucapnic and hypercapnic sleep apnea syndrome. Respiration 2008;77(2):146–53.
22. Han PY, Duffull SB, Kirkpatrick CM, et al. Dosing in obesity: a simple solution to a big problem. Clin Pharmacol Ther 2007;82(5):505–8.

23. Favetta P, Degoute CS, Perdrix JP, et al. Propofol metabolites in man following propofol induction and maintenance. Br J Anaesth 2002;88(5):653–8.
24. Cortinez LI, Anderson BJ, Penna A, et al. Influence of obesity on propofol pharmacokinetics: derivation of a pharmacokinetic model. Br J Anaesth 2010; 105(4):448–56.
25. White M, Kenny GN, Schraag S. Use of target controlled infusion to derive age and gender covariates for propofol clearance. Clin Pharmacokinet 2008;47: 119–27.
26. Dong D, Peng X, Liu J, et al. Morbid obesity alters both pharmacokinetics and pharmacodynamics of propofol: dosing recommendation for anesthesia induction. Drug Metab Dispos 2016;44(10):1579–83.
27. La Colla L, Albertin A, La Colla G, et al. No adjustment vs adjustment formula as input weight for propofol target-controlled infusion in morbidly obese patients. Eur J Anaesthesiol 2009;26(5):362–9.
28. Albertin A, Poli D, La Colla L, et al. Predictive performance of 'Servin's formula' during BIS®-guided propofol-remifentanil target-controlled infusion in morbidly obese patients. Br J Anaesth 2007;98(1):66–75.
29. Ingrande J, Lemmens HJ. Dose adjustment of anaesthetics in the morbidly obese. Br J Anaesth 2010;105(Suppl 1):i16–23.
30. Gaszynski TM, Jakubiak J, Szewczyk T. Etomidate can be dosed according to ideal body weight in morbidly obese patients. Eur J Anaesthesiol 2014;31(12): 713–4.
31. Gorlin AW, Rosenfeld DM, Ramakrishna H. Intravenous sub-anesthetic ketamine for perioperative analgesia. J Anaesthesiol Clin Pharmacol 2016;32(2):160.
32. Schwartz AE, Matteo RS, Ornstein E, et al. Pharmacokinetics and pharmacodynamics of vecuronium in the obese surgical patient. Anesth Analg 1992;74(4): 515–8.
33. Pühringer FK, Khuenl-Brady KS, Mitterschiffthaler G. Rocuronium bromide: time-course of action in underweight, normal weight, overweight and obese patients. Eur J Anaesthesiol Suppl 1995;11:107–10.
34. Pühringer FK, Keller C, Kleinsasser A, et al. Pharmacokinetics of rocuronium bromide in obese female patients. Eur J Anaesthesiol 1999;16(8):507–10.
35. Leykin Y, Pellis T, Lucca M, et al. The pharmacodynamic effects of rocuronium when dosed according to real body weight or ideal body weight in morbidly obese patients. Anesth Analg 2004;99(4):1086–9.
36. Meyhoff CS, Lund J, Jenstrup MT, et al. Should dosing of rocuronium in obese patients be based on ideal or corrected body weight? Anesth Analg 2009; 109(3):787–92.
37. Leykin Y, Pellis T, Lucca M, et al. The effects of cisatracurium on morbidly obese women. Anesth Analg 2004;99(4):1090–4.
38. Suzuki T, Masaki G, Ogawa S. Neostigmine-induced reversal of vecuronium in normal weight, overweight and obese female patients. Br J Anaesth 2006; 97(2):160–3.
39. Van Lancker P, Dillemans B, Bogaert T, et al. Ideal versus corrected body weight for dosage of sugammadex in morbidly obese patients. Anaesthesia 2011;66(8): 721–5.
40. Forman SA, Ishizawa Y. Inhaled anesthetic pharmacokinetics: uptake, distribution, metabolism and toxicity. Chapter 26. In: Miller RD, Cohen NH, Eriksson LI, et al, editors. Miller's Anesthesia. 8th edition. Elsevier; 2014. p. 638–43.
41. Lemmens HJ, Saidman LJ, Eger EI 2nd, et al. Obesity modestly affects inhaled anesthetic kinetics in humans. Anesth Analg 2008;107(6):1864–70.

42. Torri G, Casati A, Comotti L, et al. Wash-in and wash-out curves of sevoflurane and isoflurane in morbidly obese patients. Minerva Anestesiol 2002;68(6):523–7.
43. Arain SR, Barth CD, Shankar H, et al. Choice of volatile anesthetic for the morbidly obese patient: sevoflurane or desflurane. J Clin Anesth 2005;17(6): 413–9.
44. Schwartz AE, Matteo RS, Ornstein E, et al. Pharmacokinetics of sufentanil in obese patients. Anesth Analg 1991;73(6):790–3.
45. Egan TD, Huizinga B, Gupta SK, et al. Remifentanil pharmacokinetics in obese versus lean patients. Anesthesiology 1998;89(3):562–73.
46. De Baerdemaeker LE, Mortier EP, Struys MM. Pharmacokinetics in obese patients. Cont Educ Anaesth Crit Care Pain 2004;4(5):152–5.

Pharmacologic Considerations of Anesthetic Agents in Geriatric Patients

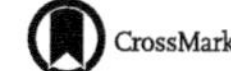

Maunak V. Rana, MD[a,*], Lara K. Bonasera, MD[a], Gregory J. Bordelon, MD[b]

KEYWORDS

- Geriatric anesthesia • Induction dosing • Pharmacokinetics
- Postoperative cognitive dysfunction (POCD) • Elderly • Aging

KEY POINTS

- Perioperative physicians should be aware of the physiologic changes with aging to avoid overdose and risk of toxicity.
- Perioperative physicians must be vigilant to the development of postoperative cognitive delirium and judiciously administer anesthetic agents in the perioperative period.
- Perioperative physicians should use a tailored approach to the anesthetic dosing of drugs because of the heterogeneity of the geriatric population.

PHARMACOLOGIC CONSIDERATIONS OF ANESTHETIC AGENTS IN GERIATRIC PATIENTS

Vigilant perioperative physicians must be cognizant of the aging population presenting for anesthetic care. Because of an increase in life expectancy coupled with improved treatments for chronic disease states, the elderly population is increasing. By 2030, 20% of the population will be older than 65 years; by 2050, 31 million citizens will be more than 80 years old.[1] Because elderly patients are 4 times more likely to undergo surgery than their younger counterparts, more procedures requiring anesthetics will result.[2,3]

Significant concerns for anesthesiologists include the development of delirium and postoperative cognitive dysfunction (POCD).[4,5] POCD and delirium are always risks in geriatric patients in the perioperative period, which mandates careful assessment of

Disclosure: The authors have nothing to disclose.

[a] Department of Anesthesiology, Advocate Illinois Masonic Medical Center, 836 West Wellington Avenue, #4815, Chicago, IL 60657, USA; [b] Department of Anesthesiology, Louisiana State University, 1542 Tulane Avenue, Room 659, New Orleans, LA 70112, USA
* Corresponding author.
E-mail address: maunakr@gmail.com

Anesthesiology Clin 35 (2017) 259–271
http://dx.doi.org/10.1016/j.anclin.2017.01.011 anesthesiology.theclinics.com
1932-2275/17/

anesthetic choices and an appreciation of the pharmacokinetics and pharmacodynamics of agents.[6,7]

Physiologic changes present in the aging population versus younger patients require perioperative physicians to be aware of the nuances of anesthetic drugs in an effort to provide an effective and structured approach to the management of geriatric patients. Age alters the pharmacokinetic and pharmacodynamic aspects of anesthetic management. The functional capacity of organs declines and coexisting diseases further contribute to physiologic decline. Awareness of age-related changes by anesthesiologists is of particular importance because of the presence of polypharmacy in elderly patients.[8] Because of the multiple drugs, which may act synergistically or at cross-purposes, the risk of adverse effects is heightened in the elderly population. It is estimated that more than 90% of persons more than 65 years of age use at least 1 drug, 40% take 5 or more drugs per week, and 12% use 10 or more drugs per week.[9,10] As a result of the potential for multiple drug interactions, a careful titration of drugs in the perioperative setting is mandated.

PHYSIOLOGIC CHANGES IN GERIATRICS

Geriatric patients share more in common with the pediatric population than younger adults because of the physiologic changes that occur in the life cycle. In general, aging is characterized by decreased reserve in organ structure and function with an increase in disorders and a decrease in homeostatic mechanisms for combating illnesses.[11] However, there is no such concept as the typical geriatric patient. This heterogeneity mandates that anesthesiologists determine where an elderly patient is on the spectrum of remarkably fit to critically ill. The changes occurring as a result of aging affect every organ system and deserve consideration (**Table 1**).

Table 1
Aging effects on organ systems/body composition in geriatric patients

Organ System	Effect
Body composition	Increased total body water: increased initial plasma volumes for bolus doses Reduced lean mass: reduced Vd of hydrophilic drugs Increased adipose tissue: increased Vd for lipophilic drugs and prolonged elimination
Renal	Decreased function Decreased renal blood flow Reduced clearance/higher serum drug levels
Hepatic	Decreased function/blood flow Decreased phase I (P450 enzyme) reactions Increased drug levels
Neurologic	Cognitive decline Decreased nerve conduction velocity Increased sensitivity to sedatives, hypnotics, opioids
Cardiac	Reduced cardiac output Increased systemic vascular resistance Reduced beta-receptor responsiveness

Abbreviation: Vd, volume of distribution.

Body Compositional Changes

Geriatric patients develop a loss in muscle mass with an increase in adipose tissue.[12,13] As a result, patients show an alteration in the volume of distribution (Vd) of anesthetic agents. The decline in muscle mass may not be readily evident because patients may have a normal creatinine value on laboratory results because of alterations in renal structure and function.[14] In contrast, there is a 20% to 40% increase in body fat with aging, which causes lipophilic agents to have a higher Vd. The net pharmacologic effect is prolonged drug action with fat-soluble agents (intravenous anesthetics).

Importantly, elderly patients also have a reduction in total body water. By age 75 years there is a 20% to 30% decline in both plasma volume and intracellular volume. The pharmacokinetic consequence of this change is a reduction in the central compartment in addition to a significant decrease in the central Vd. The net effect is a higher peak serum concentration after a bolus administration of a drug. Also, for hydrophilic agents, the plasma concentration of the agent is higher in the elderly population than in younger patients.[15]

The increased initial concentration from a bolus dose causes predictable, undesirable clinical effects. When induction doses are not reduced, exaggerated and prolonged hypotensive responses should be expected, especially with propofol.[16] Furthermore, increased initial drug levels in the central compartment, when coupled with increased circulation times from reduced myocardial performance, increase the likelihood of greater drug sensitivity and risk of toxicity.

Neurologic Structural and Functional Changes

Neurologically, there is a decrease in cerebral volume, oxygen consumption, blood flow, and blood-brain barrier permeability with aging. Losses occur in both gray and white matter, amounting to an almost 30% loss of brain mass by 80 years of age versus younger patients.[17] Findings suggest that, after 40 years, the volume and weight of the brain decline by nearly 5% per decade, and the losses accelerate once the brain reaches 70 years of age. Gender also plays a role: cerebral atrophy in men starts earlier, but develops more rapidly in women.[18]

The neuraxial space is also altered, with a reduction in cerebrospinal fluid volume, a decrease in the size of the epidural space, and an increase in dural permeability. Myelinated nerves have less myelin and also are decreased in quantity in dorsal and ventral nerve roots.[3,17,19] The net result of these changes is a decreased requirement for intravenous agents and local anesthetics, along with a lesser concentration of volatile anesthetic to achieve a desired clinical effect.

Neural processes and neurotransmitter quantity are decreased in the aging brain. In the cortex, acetylcholine receptors, serotonin receptors, and dopamine receptors decline in numbers and function with age.[17] In addition, cellular Ca^{2+} levels are altered, leading to decreased function at neuronal synapses via alteration of Ca^{2+} channel activity.

Other receptor changes with aging directly affect the administration of anesthetic agents. Changes in gamma-aminobutyric acid (GABA) receptor activity affect the actions of propofol, etomidate, and benzodiazepines. A decreased presynaptic release of GABA leads to a possible increased response by the elderly to benzodiazepines.[16]

N-Methyl-D-aspartate receptors (NMDA), involved in nociception and memory and learning, are hypofunctional with advancing age, leading to the risk of Alzheimer disease and neurodegeneration.[20] NMDA antagonists such as ketamine and dextromethorphan have the potential for altered effects in the elderly.

Nociception is altered because of the neurotransmitter and receptor changes; additionally, altered blood flow and nervous tissue damage from hyperglycemia present in the diabetic state may lead to alterations in nociception.[21]

Myocardial Structural and Functional Changes

Myocardial and vascular structure and function are altered in the elderly. Age-related changes begin as early as the fourth decade.[22] Progressive stiffening of the myocardium and vascular beds occurs primarily from cessation of elastin production, as damaged elastin is replaced by less flexible collagen.[22] There is a decrease in myocyte number and the development of concentric left ventricular hypertrophy. Functionally, these changes translate to decreased contractility, relaxation, and increased filling pressures, which are characteristic of diastolic dysfunction.[23] Increases in arterial and venous stiffness from age-related atherosclerosis, fibrosis, and calcification further contribute to myocardial hypertrophy and diastolic dysfunction. For these reasons, diastolic dysfunction is far more common than was previously appreciated, and is present in nearly one-third of elderly patients.[24]

In parallel, the autonomic nervous system is altered with aging. There is a decrease in parasympathetic function (ie, vagal tone) and an increase in sympathetic nervous system (SNS) activity. The increase in SNS activity is shown by increased circulating levels of norepinephrine coupled with decreased catecholamine uptake at nerve endings.[22] The natural consequence of increased SNS activity and vascular stiffness is the expected increase in systemic vascular resistance that is commonly seen with advancing age.

Myocardial performance is further affected by age-related alterations in the beta-adrenergic receptor activity.[22] The decline in beta-adrenergic responsiveness has several important consequences: reduced maximal attainable heart rate (chronotropy) during periods of stress and exercise (a beta-1 effect), poorer vascular relaxation (lusitropy) with direct stimulation (a beta-2 effect), and decreased myocardial contractile responsiveness (inotropy) and ejection fraction.[25] In order to meet the demands for the increased cardiac output, the aging (less compliant) myocardium relies heavily on adequate preload (intravascular volume and venous capacitance), afterload (arterial tone), and a normal sinus rhythm (atrial kick). Imbalances in these factors result in the aging myocardium being far more susceptible to failure.

Aging also degrades the myocardial conduction pathways, predisposing even the healthiest elderly patients to cardiac arrhythmias. Brady arrhythmias, heart block, and ectopic impulses coexist with beta-receptor, vascular, and diastolic dysfunction.[26]

Collectively, these alterations in beta-receptor/baroreceptor responsiveness, conduction pathway patency, myocardial relaxation, and vascular stiffness cause the blood pressure lability and orthostasis that are commonly seen in the elderly. Concomitant medications, the hypovolemic state, and anesthetic agents amplify these cardiac changes and vulnerabilities. In addition, a low cardiac output, as seen in the elderly, leads to a higher initial peak concentration because the drug is present in a smaller blood volume during injection, with a greater time to reach the target site of effect. Reduced levels of induction agents are required in the elderly, with a slower onset of action compared with younger patients.

Pulmonary

Age-related changes in the lungs and in pulmonary function occur after the third decade.[27] Because pulmonary complications account for nearly 40% of the postoperative deaths in patients more than 65 years of age, awareness of these changes is crucial.[28] The development of arthritis, kyphoscoliosis, and osteoporosis creates a less compliant thoracic cage. This stiffer chest wall increases reliance on diaphragmatic breathing, despite declining diaphragmatic strength and endurance. Faltering muscle strength and tone compromise airway protective reflexes, increasing the risk of aspiration.

Aging lung parenchyma loses elastin fibers, causing loss of elastic recoil, and altered lung volumes and capacities. This change may begin as early as the fourth decade, but naturally occurs after the fifth decade.[27] By the seventh decade, air spaces enlarge and reduce the functional alveolar surface area by 50%, causing increased compliance and functional emphysema.[27] These changes alter diffusing capacity and create V/Q mismatch, shunt, and an increased A-a gradient.[26,27] Chemoreceptor sensitivity is reduced 50% in response to hypoxia and hypercarbia.[27]

At baseline, elderly patients are noted to have lower tidal volumes and higher respiratory rates, to compensate for poorer gas exchange.[27] Taken together, all these pulmonary changes in structure, function, and mechanics predispose geriatric patients to respiratory fatigue, hypoxia, aspiration, and respiratory failure. For this reason, care must be taken to monitor for any signs of residual weakness from incompletely reversed neuromuscular blockade or sedative medications.

Renal

Changes in the renal system play a noticeable role in the metabolism and elimination of agents. Structurally, there is a 25% reduction in renal cortical mass by age 80 years, along with a decrease in renal blood flow by 10% per decade after age 40 years.[29] Further reductions in age-related renal blood flow from long-standing hypertension or diabetes predispose the aging kidney to renal dysfunction. By age 80 years, there is also a predictable 50% decrease in glomerular filtration rate (GFR), from 125 mL/min to 60 mL/min. Consequently, agents that depend on renal elimination have longer systemic half-lives and increased drug levels.[16]

Aging causes reduced renin-angiotensin function and antidiuretic hormone production, predisposing the elderly to altered volume status. As mentioned previously, serum creatinine levels are a poor predictor of renal function in older adults.[30] The GFR is the most useful value to gauge renal function.

Hepatic

Hepatic mass and blood flow decrease with aging. Liver blood flow declines 10% per decade and liver mass decreases by 35%.[31] The liver normally processes drugs via phase I and phase II reactions. Phase I reactions involve the action of the cytochrome P450 system and are slowed down by age and affected by polypharmacy. Drugs cleared by this mechanism are said to be flow limited and have a reduction in clearance of 30% to 40%, in parallel with the changes in hepatic blood flow.[32] Phase II involves the conjugation pathways, which are not affected by age. Drugs cleared primarily through this pathway are said to be capacity limited and, despite changes in hepatic mass, their clearance is well preserved, in the absence of disease, because of the presence of normal hepatic reserve.[16,32]

Protein binding

Proteins present in the plasma affect the free fraction of protein-bound drugs (most intravenous anesthetic drugs). The circulating free fraction of a drug and the free drug concentration are inversely related to plasma protein levels. Geriatric patients have lower concentrations of albumin (binds acidic drugs) because of age-related declines in production and theoretic nutritional deficits. In contrast, levels of alpha-1 acid glycoprotein, which binds basic drugs, increase only slightly with age. The clinical relevance of this effect on pharmacodynamics is not entirely predictable, and it has been suggested that it does not seem to have an important impact on geriatric anesthetic pharmacology.[33]

Plasma cholinesterase (ie, butyl cholinesterase), involved in the metabolism of succinylcholine, has decreased levels in the elderly and affects dosing of this agent.

Gastrointestinal factors

Elderly patients have increased gastric pH and also a prolonged gastric emptying time.

As a result of the physiologic changes, the geriatric patient population is at risk for overdose of agents in the perioperative period.

Pharmacokinetics/pharmacodynamics in geriatrics

In order to gain an understanding of the actions and elimination of agents in elderly patients, a brief review of pharmacologic concepts is important. The central compartment (designated as V1) is the compartment into which an agent is administered. Depending on the models being used for a particular agent, there may be 2 to 3 compartments assessed to determine pharmacokinetics. Subsequent concentrations depend on distribution and metabolism of agents into and out of the rapidly redistributed vessel-rich compartment (V2) and the vessel-poor region (V3). The total Vd is the sum of the individual compartments. Although beyond the scope of the present discussion, to evaluate the Vd of an agent, the compartment volume, redistribution, and metabolic rate constants must be considered.

Agent-specific Considerations

Induction agents

Propofol Propofol is the most commonly used induction agent. When administering this agent to elderly patients, dosage needs to be modified compared with younger patients (**Table 2**). Dosing the drug at doses that are equivalent to those of younger patients can lead to higher drug levels, which can lead to alterations in hemodynamic status.[34] In a study evaluating the pharmacokinetics of propofol in a multicenter platform, the induction doses of propofol in the elderly were as low as 1 mg/kg, far less than the conventional dose of 2 to 2.5 mg/kg in adults.[35,36] Also, the metabolic clearance of propofol declines after age 60 years. This finding was corroborated in another study that noted that propofol infusions resulted in drug concentrations that were 20% to 30% higher in geriatric patients compared with younger patients.[37] Besides the clearance effect, one study presented information on the sensitivity of geriatric patients to propofol compared with younger patients.[37] The clinical effect of propofol was measured via electroencephalogram (EEG) in adults aged 25 to 81 years and elderly patients were noted to have a 30% increased sensitivity to propofol versus younger cohorts. The investigators concluded that reductions in propofol dose as determined by the study results are not solely related to sensitivity but are also related to the altered clearance of the drug, as noted previously.[15]

Etomidate This potent induction agent is a sedative hypnotic agent with minimal hemodynamic effects when administered at induction doses. The minimal cardiovascular effects of etomidate make it a preferred agent in emergencies and for patients who cannot tolerate wide alterations in blood pressure during the induction phase of anesthesia. The drug is metabolized by ester linkage hydrolysis to inactive metabolites, which are then largely excreted in the urine. It is highly protein bound (75%), primarily to albumin.

Table 2
Effects of aging on drug behavior and dosing

Drug	Effect	Recommended Dosing Adjustments
Sedative/hypnotics	Exaggerated hypotension with bolus dosing Smaller Vd and reduced clearance	Propofol: 20%–50% reduction in bolus dosing and infusion rates Etomidate: 20%–50% reduced bolus dose
Opioids	• Increased sensitivity • Delayed renal clearance of opioid metabolites	Fentanyl/remifentanil: 50% reduction for bolus infusion rates, age>80 y Morphine, hydromorphone, meperidine: reduced doses because of concern over active metabolites
Benzodiazepines	• Increased sensitivity • Delayed renal clearance of metabolites • Increased risk for delirium/ POCD	Midazolam: reduce dose by 25%–75% Not recommended for geriatric patients
Muscle relaxants	• Delayed clearance caused by declining renal and hepatic function	Succinylcholine: no change Rocuronium: dosing intervals less frequent Cis-atracurium: no change
Inhalational agents	Minimum alveolar concentration decreases 6% per decade after age 40 y	Reduced MAC as per iso-MAC Consider BIS to guide depth

Abbreviations: BIS, bispectral index; MAC, minimal alveolar concentration.

A 50% decrease in dosage reduction is recommended in patients aged 80 years and older. The adjustment results from a reduced clearance of the drug with a decreased Vd.[38]

Ketamine The NMDA receptor antagonist ketamine is used as an induction agent and for sedation. As an antagonist to this complex, this agent shows antinociceptive effects. This agent also has a neuroprotective effect by decreasing the risk of ischemia-related apoptosis, which may lead to neuronal cell loss.[39]

Ketamine has also been advocated as an agent against POCD in elderly patients to decrease the risk of altered cognitive function after ophthalmic surgery. The recommended dose for this application is 0.3 mg/kg. This agent leads to less hypotension when given for sedation compared with propofol.[7]

Benzodiazepines The use of perioperative benzodiazepines increases the risk of postoperative delirium and should be used judiciously in geriatric patients.[40] One study evaluated midazolam, a common preoperative sedative, and noted that, after age 65 years, dosing of midazolam should be decreased compared with younger patients.[41] Midazolam clearance is reduced by 30% in 80-year-old patients compared with patients in their 20s. As a result, the dose of midazolam in geriatric patients should be decreased by at least 25%.[42] In addition, the geriatric brain is much more sensitive to midazolam, as is the case with propofol.

Dexmedetomidine Dexmedetomidine is used in for both maintenance of anesthesia and for sedation in the intensive care unit. In the elderly, the context-sensitive half-time of dexmedetomidine is prolonged and could result in prolonged sedation.

According to Iirola and colleagues,[43] 80-year-old patients have a 25% decrease in clearance compared with 60-year-olds.

Muscle relaxants/reversal agents

Succinylcholine The depolarizing neuromuscular blocker succinylcholine is used to facilitate rapid conditions for intubating patients in the perioperative period. The agent is degraded into the components succinic acid and choline by the butyl cholinesterase enzymes. With aging, levels of this plasma cholinesterase enzyme decrease; however, this alteration does not typically lead to prolonged action of succinylcholine.[44]

Rocuronium This nondepolarizing agent is primarily metabolized in the liver and excreted in the bile. Typically, rocuronium has a rapid onset of action with intermediate duration of action. Dosing of this agent is 0.45 to 1.0 mg/kg to facilitate intubating conditions and the drug has been used in maintenance states as an infusion. Although rocuronium is dosed based on ideal body weight in younger patients, elderly patients may require dose adjustment. One study evaluated the neuromuscular effects of rocuronium in elderly and younger patients, both with and without renal disease.[45] The duration of neuromuscular blockade was prolonged in elderly patients compared with younger patients for both the control group and for those patients with renal disease. A slower onset time of the agent and a prolonged duration has been compared in other studies.[46,47]

Sugammadex Sugammadex is a modified gamma-cyclodextran compound that is a selective vecuronium and rocuronium binding agent. It is biologically inactive and does not bind to plasma proteins, but to the neuromuscular blocking agents. Sugammadex is minimally metabolized, with three-fourths of the agent eliminated unchanged in the urine.[48] Rocuronium combines with sugammadex in a binding site, which leads to a decrease in the free concentration of rocuronium in the plasma.[49] In the geriatric population, sugammadex is effective in reversing neuromuscular blockade, albeit in a delayed fashion. In a phase 3a, multicenter, parallel-group, open-label study, it was noted that the time to recovery after administration of sugammadex to a train of 4 ratio of 0.9 was 3.6 minutes in geriatric patients versus 2.3 minutes in younger adults.[50] Sugammadex clearance was approximately 50% lower in the elderly patients than in younger adults. Regardless, no dose adjustment is recommended in elderly patients with normal organ function; however, because renal function is reduced in the elderly, dosing may need to be individually adjusted.[51,52]

Cisatracurium Cisatracurium is a nondepolarizing agent present as one of 10 stereoisomers of atracurium. It is 4 to 5 times more potent than atracurium, with similar duration of neuromuscular blockade, and with less histamine release.[53] This agent is eliminated via spontaneous degradation through Hoffman elimination and ester hydrolysis by plasma esterases. Hoffman elimination is a pH-dependent and temperature-dependent processes. From 77% to 80% of the drug is eliminated via Hoffman elimination; 10% to 15% is excreted unchanged in the urine.[54] In geriatric patients versus young patients, the duration of neuromuscular blockade was not altered, although the time to onset of neuromuscular blockade was delayed by 1 minute, likely because of changes in circulation time. Despite having a larger Vd compared with younger patients, the elderly patients had a minimal increase in elimination half-life. Cisatracurium clearance is unaffected by age.

Anticholinesterase agents

Anticholinesterase agents in the elderly have a theoretic risk of cardiac dysrhythmias and the presence of conduction delays. To counteract this muscarinic effect, the antimuscarinic agents are administered (preferably glycopyrrolate because there is less central effect of this agent than of the tertiary amine atropine). Some studies have noted an effect on the duration of action of neostigmine[55] versus other agents; compared with younger patients, the duration of action was prolonged in geriatric patients.[56]

Opioids Providers need to be cautious about administering opioids because effects in elders are caused by an increase in sensitivity to the agent. Risk of opioid overdose is caused by an increase in central nervous system sensitivity to opioids with age.

Fentanyl The pharmacokinetics and pharmacodynamics of this agent have been evaluated in the aging population.[57] Age was not found to have any effect on the pharmacokinetics of fentanyl. Sufentanil, alfentanil, remifentanil, and fentanyl are approximately twice as potent in elderly patients, primarily because of an increase in brain sensitivity to opioids rather than pharmacokinetic changes.[29] Except for a modest change in rapid intercompartmental clearance, the Vd is not changed compared with younger adults. The elderly brain is twice as sensitive to fentanyl and alfentanil as younger brains, although with considerable variability. As a result, providers should consider dose adjustment in geriatric perioperative patients.

Remifentanil This short-acting selective mu-receptor antagonist is typically used as an infusion for rapid analgesia because it is metabolized by nonspecific esterases. This property makes it ideal for patients with liver and/or renal dysfunction. However, the pharmacokinetics and dosing of this potent opioid require special consideration. Minto and colleagues[58,59] found that the volume of the central compartment decreased by 50% from age 20 to 80 years and the clearance decreased by 66%. As a result, age and lean body mass were determined to be important covariates affecting the pharmacokinetics of remifentanil. This finding has been corroborated elsewhere.[60] Comparing 25-year-olds and 80-year-olds getting remifentanil infusions, the clearance values are expected to decrease by 30% and central compartment values to be reduced by at least 25%.

After having established the changes in the compartments in the elderly population, the clinical effects and changes were noted compared with younger adults.[59] EEG depression as a function of sedation was noted across the age spectrum. The EC50 (effective concentration giving half-maximal response) for EEG depression decreased by approximately 50% from age 20 to 80 years. This result matched the effect of age on fentanyl potency.

Pharmacokinetic/pharmacodynamic modeling of this agent supports a 50% reduction of the bolus dose in geriatric patients versus a 20-year-old patients and a 30% to 50% reduction in infusion dosing. Elderly patients are at risk for delayed emergence without dosing adjustments.[58]

Morphine Morphine dose adjustment needs to occur because of multiple factors. Morphine is processed by conjugation in the liver to morphine-3 glucuronide and morphine-6 glucuronide. Morphine-3 glucuronide is a neurotoxic agent that can lead to seizures. Morphine-6 glucuronide has analgesic properties. Both are renally cleared and have decreased clearance in the elderly.[61]

Inhaled agents

Perioperative physicians also need to consider unique factors in the geriatric population when adjusting inhaled anesthetic concentrations. The minimal alveolar concentration (MAC) to surgical stimulus decreases by 6% for every decade of life.[62] Currently used agents are considered individually, with unique considerations for each agent. In addition, the use of iso-MAC scales is used to allow for the addition of nitrous-oxide/oxygen to inhaled potent agents. End-expired agent in terms of MAC is graphed versus age of subject and data points presented for End-expired agent in 100% oxygen, 67% nitrous oxide and 50 % nitrous oxide.[63]

Sevoflurane Sevoflurane is perhaps the most commonly used agent for maintenance of inhaled anesthesia. The MAC for sevoflurane was noted to be 1.48, decreased from children and adults, with a calculated ED95 (the effective dose required to prevent 95% of patients from moving) of 1.98%.[64] This age-related change in dosage of sevoflurane is corroborated by the finding of midlatency auditory evoked potentials (MLAEPs) as a marker for anesthetic depth. Elderly patients need lower anesthetic concentrations of sevoflurane than younger patients to achieve a similar MLAEP level.[65] It has been evaluated as an agent for inhaled inductions in ambulatory geriatric patients compared with propofol induction. The sevoflurane inhaled induction patients were noted to have less alteration in mean arterial pressure and systolic pressure versus their propofol cohorts. This finding would lead to fewer instances of hemodynamic alteration for the induction phase of anesthesia.[66]

Another study evaluated sevoflurane induction in patients undergoing esophageal resection to assess for any effects on POCD in patients receiving sevoflurane anesthesia. Patients were placed into sevoflurane inhaled anesthesia, sevoflurane with preoperative methylprednisolone before potent agent, and intravenous propofol control.[4] Cognitive assessment was performed before surgery and on days 1, 3, and 7 postoperatively along with evaluation for inflammatory and neurocognitive markers. The results indicated that the incidence of POCD was higher in patients under inhalational sevoflurane than in the other groups. Methylprednisolone was a salubrious pretreatment neuroprotective agent. Although these results are singular, for more invasive operations that may be time laborious, a multimodal regimen is advocated for neuroprotection.

Desflurane This insoluble inhaled anesthetic allows rapid redistribution and wake up with maintenance of potent anesthesia. For the geriatric population, a decrease in MAC is determined for geriatric patients, down to 5.1% for 80-year-old patients versus 8.3% in adults. This is an important consideration given the risk of tachycardia that can occur with rapid increases in anesthetic concentration of desflurane.

Isoflurane This agent has been used less because of the increased use of sevoflurane and desflurane. In the elderly, isoflurane decreases systemic pressure, cardiac index, and heart rate.

REFERENCES

1. Day JC. Population projections of the United States by age, sex, race, and Hispanic origin: 1995-2050, current population reports, Bureau of the Census. Washington, DC: US Printing Office; 1996. p. 25.
2. Cook DJ, Rooke GA. Priorities in perioperative geriatrics. Anesth Analg 2003;96: 1823–36.
3. Brown EN, Purdon PL. The aging brain and anesthesia. Curr Opin Anaesthesiol 2013;26:414–9.
4. Qiao Y, Feng H, Zhao T, et al. Postoperative cognitive dysfunction after inhalational anesthesia in elderly patients undergoing major surgery: the influence of anesthetic technique, cerebral injury and systemic inflammation. BMC Anesthesiol 2015;15:154.

5. Deiner S, Silverstein JH. Postoperative delirium and cognitive dysfunction. Br J Anaesth 2009;103(Suppl 1):i41–6.
6. Rundshagen I. Postoperative cognitive dysfunction. Dtsch Arztebl Int 2014 Feb; 111(8):119–25.
7. Rascon-Martinez DM, Fresan-Orellana A, Ocharan-Hernandez ME, et al. The effects of ketamine on cognitive function in elderly patients undergoing ophthalmic surgery: a pilot study. Anesth Analg 2016;122(4):969–75.
8. Wehling M. Guideline-driven polypharmacy in elderly, multimorbid patients is basically flawed: there are almost no guidelines for these patients. J Am Geriatr Soc 2011;59:376–7.
9. Qato DM, Alexander GC, Conti RM, et al. Use of prescription and over-the-counter medication and dietary supplements among older adults in the United States. JAMA 2008;300:2867–78.
10. Gurwitz JH, Field TS, Harrold LR, et al. Incidence and preventability of adverse drug event among older persons in the ambulatory setting. JAMA 2003;289: 1107–16.
11. Shafer S. Challenges in anesthesia: The geriatric patient presenting for surgery. Chapter 50. In: Chu LF, Fuller AJ, editors. Manual of clinical anesthesiology. 1st edition. Philadelphia: Lippincott Williams & Wilkins; 2012.
12. Forbes GB, Reina JC. Adult lean body mass declines with age: some longitudinal observations. Metabolism 1970;19:653–63.
13. Beaufrere B, Morio B. Fat and protein redistribution with aging: metabolic considerations. Eur J Clin Nutr 2000;3(Suppl 54):S48–53.
14. Cockcroft DW, Gault MH. Prediction of creatinine clearance from serum creatinine. Nephron 1976;16:31–41.
15. Shafer SL. The pharmacology of anesthetic drugs in elderly patients. Anesthesiol Clin North America 2000;18:1–29.
16. Spanjer MRK, Bakker NA, Absalom AR. Pharmacology in the elderly and newer anaesthesia drugs. Best Pract Res Clin Anaesthesiol 2011;25:355–65.
17. Peters R. Ageing and the brain. Postgrad Med J 2006;82:84–8.
18. Small SA. Age-related memory decline: current concepts and future directions. Arch Neurol 2001;58:360–4.
19. Sieber FE, Pauldine R. Anesthesia for the elderly. In: Miller's anesthesia. 7th edition. Philadelphia: Elsevier Churchill Livingstone; 2010. p. 2261–76.
20. Newcomer JW, Farber NB. NMDA receptor function, memory and brain aging. Dialogues Clin Neurosci 2000;2(3):219–32.
21. McKeown JL. Pain management issues for the geriatric surgical patient. Anesthesiology Clin 2015;33:563–76.
22. Rooke GA. Cardiovascular aging and the anesthetic implications. J Cardiothorac Vasc Anesth 2003;17:512–23.
23. Steppan J, Barodka V, Berkowitz DE, et al. Vascular stiffness and increases pulse pressure in the aging cardiovascular system. Cardiol Res Pract 2011;2011:263585.
24. Bursi F, Weston SA, Redfield MM, et al. Systolic and diastolic heart failure in the community. JAMA 2006;296:2209–16.
25. Priebe HJ. The aged cardiovascular risk patient. Br J Anaesth 2000;85:763–8.
26. Kanonidou Z, Karystianou G. Anesthesia for the elderly. Hippokratia 2007;11(4): 175–7.
27. Sprung J, Gajic O, Warner DO. Review article: age related alterations in respiratory function–anesthetic considerations. Can J Aneaesth 2006;53(12):1244–57.
28. Warner DO. Preventing postoperative pulmonary complications. Anesthesiology 2000;92:1467–72.

29. Brown CH, Sieber F. The elderly patient. Chapter 21. In: McConachie I, editor. Anesthesia and perioperative care of the high-risk patient. 3rd edition. Cambridge University Press, Cambridge University; 2014. p. 311–22.
30. Musso CG, Oreopoulos DG. Aging and physiological changes of the kidneys including changes in glomerular filtration rate. Nephron Physiol 2011;119:1–5.
31. McLean AJ, LeCouteur DG. Aging biology and geriatric clinical pharmacology. Pharmacol Rev 2004;56:163–84.
32. Rivera R, Antognini JF. Perioperative drug therapy in elderly patients. Anesthesiology 2009;10(5):1176–89.
33. Benet LZ, Hoener BA. Changes in plasma protein binding have little clinical relevance. Clin Pharmacol Ther 2002;71:115–21.
34. Kazama T, Ikeda K, Morita K. Reduction by fentanyl of the CP50 values of propofol and hemodynamic responses to various noxious stimuli. Anesthesiology 1997; 87(2):213–27.
35. Schuttler J, Ihmsen H. Population pharmacokinetics of propofol: a multicenter study. Anesthesiology 2000;92(3):727–38.
36. Schnider TW, Minto CF, Shafer SL, et al. The influence of the method of administration and covariates on the pharmacokinetic of propofol in adults volunteers. Anesthesiology 1998;43(Suppl):111–4.
37. Schnider TW, Minto CF, Shafer SL, et al. The influence of age on propofol pharmacodynamics. Anesthesiology 1999;90(6):1502–16.
38. Arden JR, Holley FO, Stanski DR. Increased sensitivity to etomidate in the elderly: initial distribution versus altered brain response. Anesthesiology 1986;65:19–27.
39. Engelhard K, Werner C, Eberspacher E, et al. The effect of the alpha-2 agonist dexmedetomidine and N-methyl-D-Aspartate antagonist S (+) ketamine on the expression of apoptosis-regulating proteins after incomplete cerebral ischemia and reperfusion in rats. Anesth Analg 2003;96:524–31.
40. Marcantonio ER, Juarez G, Goldman L, et al. The relationship of postoperative delirium with psychoactive medications. JAMA 1994;272:1518–22.
41. Bell GD, Spickett GP, Reeve PA, et al. Intravenous midazolam for upper gastrointestinal endoscopy: a study of 800 consecutive cases relating dose to age and sex of patient. Br J Clin Parmacol 1987;23:241–3.
42. Maitre PO, Buhrer M, Thomson D, et al. A three-step approach combining Bayesian regression and NONMEM population analysis: application to midazolam. J Pharmacokinet Biopharm 1991;19:377–84.
43. Iirola T, Ihmsen H, Laitio R, et al. Population pharmacokinetics of dexmedetomidine during long-term sedation in intensive care patients. Br J Anaesth 2012; 108(3):460–8.
44. Cope TM, Hunter JM. Selecting neuromuscular-blocking drugs for elderly patients. Drugs Aging 2003;20(2):125–40.
45. Kocabas S, Yedicocuklu D, Askar FZ. The neuromuscular effects of rocuronium in elderly and young adults with or without renal failure: 9AP7-7. Eur J Anaesthesiol 2007;24:124.
46. Matteo RS, Ornstein E, Schwartz AE, et al. Pharmacokinetics and pharmacodynamics of rocuronium (Org 9426) in elderly surgical patients. Anesth Analg 1993;77:1193–7.
47. Furuya T, Suzuki T, Kashiwai A, et al. The effects of age on maintenance of intense neuromuscular block with rocuronium. Acta Anaesthesiol Scand 2012;56:236–9.
48. Gijsenbergh R, Ramael S, Houwing N, et al. First human exposure of Org 25969, a novel agent to reverse the action of rocuronium bromide. Anesthesiology 2005; 103:695–703.

49. Mirakhur RK. Sugammadex in clinical practice. Anesthesiology 2009;64(Suppl 1): 45–54.
50. McDonagh DL, Benedict PE, Kovac AL, et al. Efficacy, safety and pharmacokinetics of sugammadex for the reversal of rocuronium-induced neuromuscular blockade in elderly patients. Anesthesiology 2011;114:318–29.
51. Merck & Co Bridion (sugammadex) injection, for intravenous use: US prescribing information. 2015. Available at: http://www.accessdata.fda.gov/. Accessed June 8, 2016.
52. European Medicines Agency. Bridion (sugammadex) 100mg/mL solution for injection: EU summary of product characteristics. 2015. Available at: http://www.ema.europa.eu/. Accessed June 8, 2016.
53. Ornstein E, Lien CA, Matteo RS, et al. Pharmacodynamics and pharmacokinetics of cisatracurium in geriatric surgical patients. Anesthesiology 1996;84:520–5.
54. Appiah-Ankam J, Hunter JM. Pharmacology of neuromuscular blocking drugs. Contin Educ Anaesth Crit Care Pain 2004;4(1):2–7.
55. Koscielniak-Nielsen ZJ, Law-Min JC, Donati F, et al. Dose-response relations of doxacurium and its reversal with neostigmine in young adults and healthy elderly patients. Anesth Analg 1992;74(6):845–50.
56. Young WL, Matteo RS, Ornstein E. Duration of action of neostigmine and pyridostigmine in the elderly. Anesth Analg 1988;67(8):775–8.
57. Scott JC, Stanski DR. Decreased fentanyl and alfentanil dose requirements with age. A simultaneous pharmacokinetic and pharmacodynamic evaluation. J Pharmacol Exp Ther 1987;240:159–66.
58. Minto CF, Schnider TW, Egan T, et al. The influence of age and gender on the pharmacokinetics and pharmacodynamics of remifentanil. I. Model development. Anesthesiology 1997;86:10–23.
59. Minto CF, Schnider TW, Shafer SL. The influence of age and gender on the pharmacokinetic and pharmacodynamics of remifentanil. II. Model application. Anesthesiology 1997;86:24–33.
60. Glass PS, Gan TJ, Howell S. A review of the pharmacokinetics and pharmacodynamics of remifentanil. Anesth Analg 1999;89(Suppl 4):S7–14.
61. Baillie SP, Bateman DN, Coates PE, et al. Age and the pharmacokinetics of morphine. Age Ageing 1989;18:258–62.
62. Eger E. Age, minimum alveolar anesthetic concentration, and minimum alveolar anesthetic concentration-awake. Anesth Analg 2001;93:947–53.
63. Nickalls RWD, Mapleson WW. Age-related iso-MAC charts for isoflurane, sevoflurane and desflurane in man. Br J Anaesth 2003;91(2):170–4.
64. Nakajima R, Nakajima Y, Ikeda K. Minimum alveolar concentration of sevoflurane in elderly patients. Br J Anaesth 1993;70(3):273–5.
65. Feuerecker M, Lenk M, Flake G, et al. Effects of increasing sevoflurane MAC levels on mid-latency auditory evoked potentials in infants, schoolchildren, and the elderly. Br J Anaesth 2011;107(5):726–34.
66. Kirkbride DA, Parker JL, Williams GD, et al. Induction of anesthesia in the elderly ambulatory patient: a double-blinded comparison of propofol and sevoflurane. Anesth Analg 2001;93:1185–7.

Cardiovascular Pharmacology

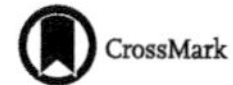

An Update and Anesthesia Considerations

Camellia Asgarian, MD[a,*], Henry Liu, MD[b],
Alan D. Kaye, MD, PhD, DABA, DABPM, DABIPP[a]

KEYWORDS

• Cardiovascular • Pharmacology • Anesthesia • Hemodynamic instability

KEY POINTS

- Cardiovascular disease remains a leading cause of morbidity and mortality, not only in the United States but it is also increasing as a leading cause of death worldwide.
- The development of therapeutic agents for the treatment of cardiovascular diseases has always been a priority for the pharmaceutical industry because of the huge potential market for these drugs.
- These medications should be part of the anesthesiologist's armamentarium because the typical surgical patient is older and has more comorbidities than in the past.
- This article reviews commonly used cardiovascular medications that are important in managing a patient with unstable hemodynamics.

INTRODUCTION

Cardiovascular disease remains a leading cause of morbidity and mortality, not only in the United States but it is also increasing as a leading cause of death worldwide.[1–6] The development of therapeutic agents for the treatment of cardiovascular diseases has always been a priority for the pharmaceutical industry because of the huge potential market for these drugs. These medications should be part of the anesthesiologist's armamentarium because the typical surgical patient is older and has more comorbidities than in the past (**Table 1**). This article reviews commonly used cardiovascular medications that are important in managing a patient with unstable hemodynamics.

[a] Department of Anesthesiology, LSU School of Medicine, T6M5, 1542 Tulane Avenue, Room 656, New Orleans, LA 70112, USA; [b] Department of Anesthesiology & Perioperative Medicine, Hahnemann University Hospital, Drexel University College of Medicine, 245 North 15th Street, MS 310, Philadelphia, PA 19102, USA
* Corresponding author.
E-mail address: casgar@lsuhsc.edu

Anesthesiology Clin 35 (2017) 273–284
http://dx.doi.org/10.1016/j.anclin.2017.01.013 anesthesiology.theclinics.com
1932-2275/17/

Table 1
New York Heart Association classification for heart failure patients based on symptoms

NYHA Class	Patients' Symptoms
Class I (mild)	No limitation of physical activity. Ordinary physical activity does not cause undue fatigue, palpitation, or dyspnea
Class II (mild)	Slight limitation of physical activity, comfortable at rest but ordinary physical activity results in fatigue, palpitation, or dyspnea
Class III (moderate)	Marked limitation of physical activity, comfortable at rest but less than ordinary activity causes fatigue, palpitation, or dyspnea
Class IV (severe)	Unable to carry out physical activity without discomfort. Symptoms of cardiac insufficiency at rest. If any physical activity is undertaken, discomfort is increased

From The Criteria Committee of the New York Heart Association. Nomenclature and criteria for diagnosis of diseases of the heart and great vessels. 9th edition. Boston: Little, Brown & Co; 1994. p. 253–6; with permission.

ANATOMY OF CARDIAC MUSCLE FIBER AND SARCOMERES

Human muscles are categorized into 3 types: skeletal, cardiac, and smooth muscle. The cells that form cardiac muscles are called cardiomyocytes and are striated, involuntary muscles. They are sometimes seen as an intermediate between the other 2 types of muscles in terms of appearance, structure, metabolism, excitation coupling, and mechanism of contraction. Cardiac muscle shares some similarities with skeletal muscle in its striated appearance and contraction, and both are multinuclear compared with the mononuclear smooth muscle cells.[7] However, the myofibrils of cardiac muscle cells may be branched instead of linear and longitudinal as in skeletal muscle cells. These branches interlock with those of adjacent fibers by adherens junctions. These strong junctions enable the heart to contract forcefully without ripping the fibers apart. Also, the T-tubules in cardiac muscle are larger, broader, and run along the Z disks. The cardiac muscles contain fewer T-tubules compared with skeletal muscle. T-tubules play a critical role in excitation-contraction coupling (ECC).[7]

The primary structural proteins of cardiac muscle are actin and myosin. As shown in **Fig. 1**, the actin filaments are thin, causing the lighter appearance represented by I-bands in striated muscle (see **Fig. 1**A); the thicker myosin filament is represented by a darker appearance to the alternating A-bands observed microscopically (see **Fig. 1**B). The A-bands are bisected by the H-zone, with the M-line running through the center. The H-zone is that portion of the A-band where there is no overlap between the thick and thin bands. The I-bands are bisected by the Z-disk. Each myofibril is made up of arrays of parallel filaments. The thin filaments are primarily composed of actin along with smaller amounts of 2 other proteins: troponin (TN) and tropomyosin. The thick filaments have a diameter of 15 to 20 nm (see **Fig. 1**D). They are composed of the protein myosin. The array of thick and thin filaments between the Z-disks is called a sarcomere. Molecules of a giant protein, titin (2500 kDa), extend from the M-line to the Z-disk and are closely associated with the myosin molecule. They seem to anchor the myosin network to the actin network and maintain the neatly ordered striation pattern. One of its functions is to provide a scaffold for the assembly of a precise number of myosin molecules in the thick filament. Titin may also dictate the number of actin molecules in the thin filaments. In a myofibril, shortening of the sarcomeres shortens the myofibril and the muscle fibers. Cardiac myosin is the motor

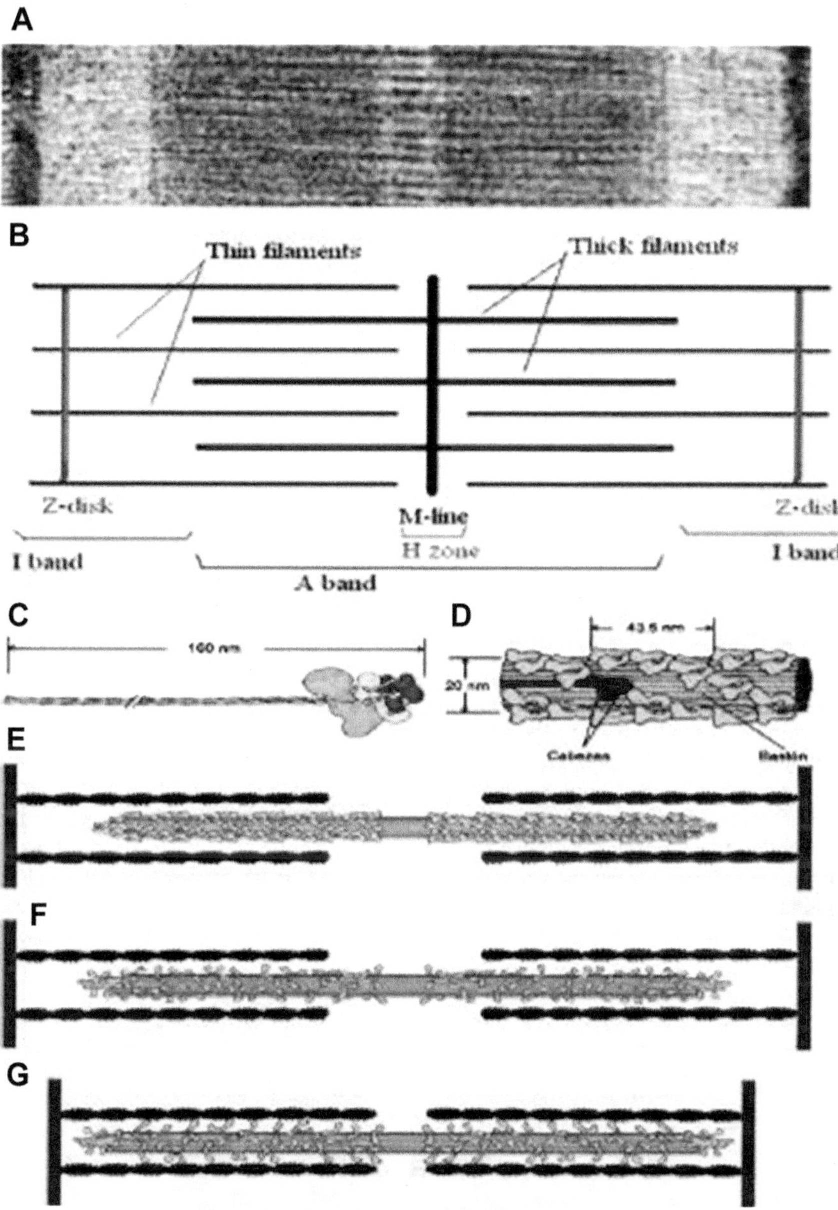

Fig. 1. (*A–G*) The structure of myofibril, the basic functional unit of striated muscle. ([*A, B*] *Courtesy of* H. Liu, MD, New Orleans, LA; and [*C–G*] *Adapted from* Padrón R. El modelo atómico del filamento de miosina. Investigación y Ciencia 2007; with permission.)

protein directly responsible for converting chemical energy into the mechanical force that results in cardiac contraction. When the muscle is relaxed, myosin and actin are not engaged (see **Fig. 1**E). However, when the sarcomere is activated and contracting (see **Fig. 1**F), the myosin and actin proteins are engaged, and the sarcomere is shortened (see **Fig. 1**G). Cardiac contractility is driven by the cardiac sarcomere. The sarcomere is among the most thoroughly characterized protein machines in human biology.

EXCITATION-CONTRACTION COUPLING: THE CARDIAC ACTION POTENTIAL

An action potential (AP) originating in the sinus node depolarizes the cardiomyocyte and calcium ion enters the cytoplasm in phase 2 of the AP through L-type calcium channel, which is located on the sarcolemma. The intracellular calcium then triggers the subsequent release of calcium that is stored in sarcoplasmic reticulum (SR) through calcium-releasing channels. The binding of free calcium to TN-C, part of the regulatory protein complex attached to the thin filaments, induces a conformational change in the regulatory complex such that TN-I exposes a site on the actin molecule that is able to bind to the myosin adenosine triphosphatase (ATPase) located on the myosin head (**Fig. 2**). This binding results in adenosine triphosphate (ATP) hydrolysis, which supplies energy for a conformational change to occur in the actin-myosin complex. This results in movement (ratcheting) between the myosin heads and the actin, such that the actin and myosin filaments slide past each other and shorten the sarcomere length. Ratcheting cycles occur as long as the cytosolic calcium remains increased. At the end of phase 2, calcium entry into the cell slows and calcium is sequestered by the SR by an ATP-dependent calcium pump (sarcoendoplasmic reticulum calcium-ATPase), which lowers the cytosolic calcium concentration and removes calcium from the TN-C. To a lesser extent, cytosolic calcium is transported out of the cell by the sodium-calcium exchange pump. The reduced intracellular calcium induces a conformational change in the TN complex, leading to TN-I inhibition of the actin-binding site. This inhibition disengages the myosin head and actin-binding site. At the end of the cycle, a new ATP binds to the myosin head, displacing the adenosine diphosphate, and the initial sarcomere length is restored. If the cytosolic calcium level cannot reach the necessary level, cardiac systolic function will be compromised. However, if the cytoplasmic calcium level is unable to reach the lower resting level, cardiac diastolic dysfunction will occur.

The calcium ion plays a critically important role in ECC in the myocardium. Most inotropes used to treat congestive heart failure increase the intracellular calcium level. β-Adrenergic receptor agonist or phosphodiesterase inhibitor (PDE-i) achieves

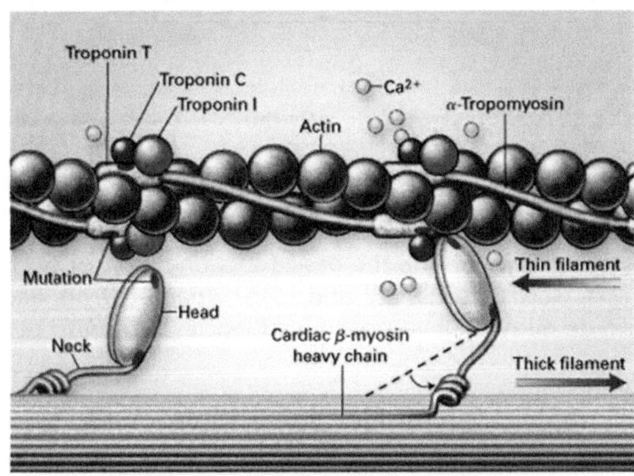

Fig. 2. Sliding filament theory of contraction. (*From* Kamisago M, Sharma SD, DePalma SR, et al. Mutations in sarcomere protein genes as a cause of dilated cardiomyopathy. N Engl J Med 2000;343(23):1688–96; with permission.)

increased myocardial contractility by increasing the delivery of intracellular calcium to the sarcomeres through increasing the intracellular level of cyclic adenosine monophosphate (cAMP) (**Fig. 3**). However, evidence suggests that this pathway may lead to adverse clinical outcomes. Current inotropic therapy (catecholamines, PDE-i) was associated with a 2-fold increase in the risk of in-hospital mortality compared with treatment with vasodilators. In-hospital mortalities were 12.3% and 13.9% in patients receiving milrinone or dobutamine versus 4.7% and 7.1% in those receiving nitrates or nesiritide, respectively.[8] Fellahi and colleagues[9–13] studied 657 subjects, 84 (13%) of whom received catecholamines, most often dobutamine (76 of 84, 90%). A higher incidence of both major cardiac morbidity (30% vs 9%) and all-cause intrahospital mortality (8% vs 1%) was observed in the catecholamine group compared with the control group. After adjusting for channeling bias and confounding factors, catecholamine administration was significantly associated with major cardiac morbidity after propensity score stratification, propensity score covariance analysis, marginal structural models, and propensity score matching but not with all-cause intrahospital mortality. The potential mechanism behind these worse than expected results in the catecholamine-treated group may be the increased velocity of the cardiac contraction, which shortens systolic ejection time.

DRUGS FOR THE MANAGEMENT OF HEMODYNAMIC INSTABILITY

Hemodynamic instability occurs when the patient's blood pressure (BP) and heart rate are greater than 40% outside normal values, or when the mean arterial pressure (MAP) is less than 65 mm Hg or greater than 120 mm Hg. This can occur for a multitude of

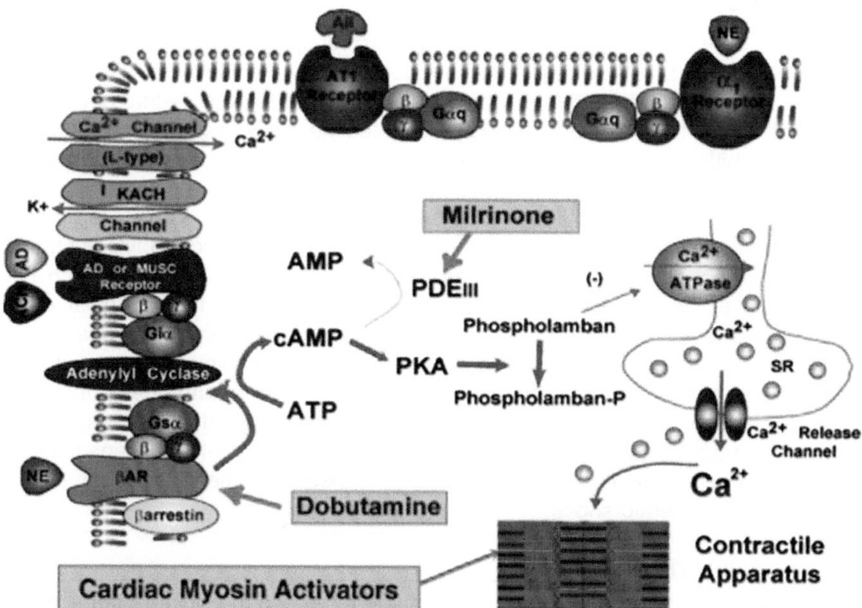

Fig. 3. Myocyte and signaling pathways. ACH, acetylcholine; AD, adenosine; AMP, adenosine monophosphate; ATP, adenosine triphosphate; cAMP, cyclic adenosine monophosphate; CA^{2+}, calcium; MUSC, muscarinic; NE, norepinephrine; PDE, phosphodiesterase; PKA, protein kinase A; βAR, beta adrenergic receptor. (*From* Teerlink JR. A novel approach to improve cardiac performance: cardiac myosin activators. Heart Fail Rev 2009;14:291; with permission.)

reasons, ranging from the anesthetic dosing or volume status to life-threatening conditions such as a myocardial infarction or circulatory shock. Hemodynamic instability is more likely to be encountered in certain situations, such as weaning from cardiopulmonary bypass. The pharmacologic management in these situations is generally the responsibility of the anesthesiologist and knowledge of the following drugs is essential.

VASOPRESSORS

Vasopressin

Vasopressin, also known as arginine vasopressin and antidiuretic hormone, is a unique vasopressor in that it functions through a different set of receptors and pathways than the catecholamine vasopressor and inotropic agents. Vasopressin is an endogenous hormone formed in the posterior pituitary gland. Its actions are mediated through numerous G-protein coupled receptors, the most important of which are the V_1 (vascular) and V_2 (renal) subtypes. The V_1 receptors are found in a wide variety of tissues, including vascular smooth muscle, the kidneys, platelets, and cardiomyocytes. Its effect on vascular smooth muscle is vasoconstriction, which is the most immediate way in which it increases BP. However, although it functions as an antidiuretic and can increase fluid retention via activation of the V_2 receptor, vasopressin also increases glomerular filtration in the kidneys and paradoxically may increase urine output via activation of V_1 receptors in the kidney. Vasopressin does not affect the pulmonary vasculature and is generally favored for treating hypotension in the setting of right heart failure because it does not increase the afterload on the right heart.

Methylene Blue

Methylene blue is an agent generally used as a last resort in patients with severe vasodilatory shock refractory to other pressor agents. It has many uses in the operating room: as a treatment of methemoglobinemia, to help identify the ureters or parathyroid gland, and to treat the vasoplegic patient. Methylene blue exerts its vasopressor effect by inhibiting the action of nitric oxide (NO) synthase and thus decreasing the production of NO. A hypertensive response is generally not seen in hemodynamically stable patients receiving methylene blue because it simply reduces the responsiveness of blood vessels to NO and other vasodilators that act through NO synthase. Methylene blue can be administered as a single dose (1.5–2 mg/kg), which has been shown to be effective, or as a maintenance infusion after an initial bolus dose. Studies looking at the efficacy of methylene blue show that it decreases the dose and duration of use of other vasoconstrictors to maintain an adequate perfusion pressure. It is, however, best used in a truly vasoplegic patient and does not reliably restore systemic vascular resistance (SVR) in patients with hypotension due to other factors. The most common situations that may necessitate use of methylene blue are in cardiac surgery patients postbypass, in liver transplant patients postreperfusion, and in patients in septic shock.

Intravenous Antihypertensive Drugs

Approximately 72 million people suffer from hypertension in the United States, which accounts for almost a third of the adult population. Hypertension is among the most common chronic medical conditions in adult Americans. Hypertension affects more men than women, and almost twice as many African Americans as whites. The incidence of hypertension increases with age. Management of patients with chronic hypertension undergoing surgery is of major clinical importance because they experience an increased risk of morbidity and mortality after surgery. When managing patients with hypertensive crisis in the emergency room, it is ideal to have drugs that possess the following features: fast-onset, short-acting, predictable dose responses, minimal titration time to desired BP, fewer dose adjustments, fewer adverse effects, no effect on intracranial pressure, no cerebral or coronary steal, no negative effect on cardiac contractility and conduction, and no reliance on renal or hepatic function for their clearance. Although no such drug is available, several newer drugs, such as nicardipine and clevidipine, possess many desirable characteristics.

Nicardipine

Nicardipine hydrochloride (Cardene) is a calcium ion influx inhibitor (slow channel blocker or calcium channel blocker). Its structure is shown in **Fig. 4**. Nicardipine hydrochloride is a greenish-yellow, odorless, crystalline powder that is freely soluble in chloroform, methanol, and glacial acetic acid. Its dose response is linear from 0.5 to 40 mg/h. Its rapid early distribution phase (a) half time is 2.7 minutes, intermediate phase (b) half time is 44.8 minutes, and its slow terminal phase (g) half time is 14.4 hours. Nicardipine is metabolized in the liver by P450 3A2. The onset time of nicardipine is 1 minute and peak time is 5 to 10 minutes after intravenous administration. Currently, nicardipine is available for both oral and intravenous formulations. Hydrochloric acid and/or sodium hydroxide may have been added to adjust pH to between 3.7 and 4.7. If intravenous nicardipine is administered through a peripheral venous catheter, it may necessitate changing the venous site after a couple of days because of its potent venous irritant effect.

Nicardipine intravenous administration has been compared with sodium nitroprusside (believed to be the gold standard of antihypertensive drugs) for hypertensive therapy after coronary artery bypass graft (CABG) surgery. Within 6 hours after surgery, 47 subjects after CABG, with systolic BP (SBP) of 150 mm Hg or greater, were randomized to receive either intravenous nicardipine or sodium nitroprusside. Both drugs were infused at 2 mg/kg/min for 10 minutes. The dosage was increased by 1 mg/kg/min every 10 minutes if the BP remained higher than the target BP and was decreased by 1 mg/kg/min when the target BP was achieved. No differences in SBP or heart rate were reported but the duration of drug therapy and the total dose administered were lower for the nicardipine group compared with the sodium nitroprusside group. Cardiac index and stroke volume were higher and SVR was lower in patients treated with nicardipine.[14] Nicardipine has also been used to treat cardiac diastolic dysfunction and it is used to prevent spasm of arterial graft for coronary artery bypass. The side effects of nicardipine include headache (14.6%), hypotension (5.6%), nausea and vomiting (4.9%), and tachycardia (3.5%).

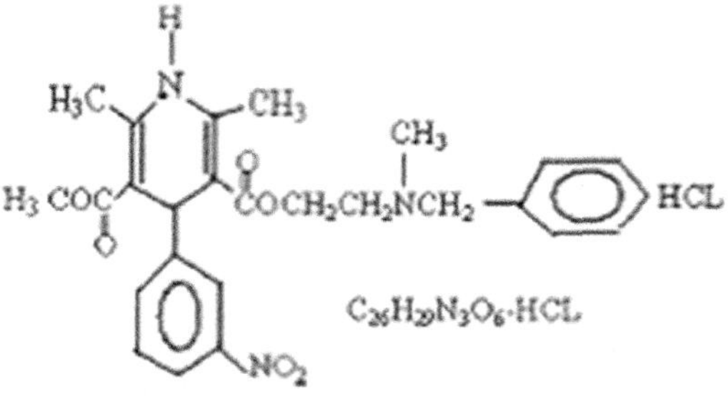

Fig. 4. Nicardipine hydrochloride. (*Courtesy of* H. Liu, MD, New Orleans, LA.)

Clevidipine

Clevidipine (Cleviprex) is a vasoselective, ultra–short-acting, third-generation dihydropyridine L-type calcium channel blocker. It was approved on August 4, 2008 by the US Food and Drug Administration (FDA) for the reduction of BP when oral therapy is not feasible or desirable. Clevidipine is selective for arteriolar vasodilatation; thus, it lowers MAP by decreasing SVR without reducing cardiac filling pressures. It produces little or no effect on myocardial contractility or cardiac conduction, a potentially favorable feature in patients after cardiac surgery. Clevidipine's selectivity for arterial vessels allows a direct reduction in peripheral vascular resistance without dilatation of the venous capacitance bed. Clevidipine is similar in structure to felodipine, an oral vasoselective dihydropyridine calcium channel antagonist, with the exception of an additional ester linkage that is responsible for its rapid metabolism.

Clevidipine is a racemic mixture of 2 enantiomers, S-clevidipine and R-clevidipine. Like other dihydropyridine calcium channel antagonists, clevidipine exerts its effects by inhibiting transmembrane calcium influx through voltage-dependent L-type calcium channels with a high degree of vascular selectivity for arterial smooth muscle and no effect on venous capacitance vessels. Clevidipine is 3 to 6 times more potent at the lower resting membrane potentials that are seen in vascular smooth muscle, compared with cardiac myocytes that show a greater negative resting membrane potential. Because of this, the effect of clevidipine on myocardial contractility is limited.[15–17] A decrease in BP is observed within 2 to 3 minutes after intravenous administration of clevidipine. The BP returns to pretreatment levels within 5 to 15 minutes of terminating the infusion, primarily as a result of the drug's high clearance rate (0.13 L/min/kg) and small volume of distribution at steady state (0.6 L/kg), resulting in an initial phase half-life of approximately 1 minute and terminal phase half-life of 10 to 15 minutes. In studies of up to 72 hours of continuous infusion, there was no evidence of tolerance. At steady state, arterial blood concentration of clevidipine is twice that of venous blood, which results in an increased clearance rate (0.05 L/min/kg) and a smaller volume of distribution (0.17 L/kg). These arteriovenous concentration differences have also been observed in other short-acting compounds containing an ester linkage in their structure. More than 80% of the total area under the blood concentration-time curve is associated with the initial phase half-life owing to rapid elimination of drug rather than distribution, as is evident from postinfusion blood concentrations that decrease by 50% within 1 minute of stopping the infusion, regardless of the duration. Clevidipine is rapidly metabolized by esterases in the blood and extravascular tissues and, as such, it is unlikely to be affected by renal or hepatic insufficiency. Even in patients with pseudocholinesterase deficiency, it is rapidly metabolized. The major route of elimination is via the kidney, with 63% to 73% of radioactively labeled clevidipine recovered in the urine, and 10% to 20% recovered in the feces. Because of the lack of hepatic metabolism, clevidipine is not expected to be affected by changes in cytochrome P450 isoenzyme activity. The drug is highly protein bound (99.5%) in human plasma, in a non–concentration-dependent manner, and binding to specific plasma proteins, such as A-1-acid glycoprotein, has not been elucidated. Clevidipine is contraindicated in patients with severe aortic stenosis; severe hypertrophic obstructive cardiomyopathy; or allergies to soybeans, soy products, eggs, or egg products.

Inotropes and Inodilators

Little has changed in regard to inotropic therapy over the past few decades. The beta-adrenergic agonists (epinephrine, norepinephrine, dobutamine) are generally favored for the treatment of cardiogenic shock and acute decompensated systolic heart failure. Milrinone is a phosphodiesterase-3 (PDE-3) inhibitor that causes an increase in intracellular cAMP levels in cardiac myocytes and a subsequent increase in intracellular calcium levels. Milrinone is best used for patients in acute systolic heart failure with pulmonary hypertension, patients requiring beta blockade or patients with normal renal function. Despite the widespread use of all of these medications, data have shown that the use of positive inotropic agents causes increased morbidity and mortality. The main complications from inotropes are arrhythmias, induced myocardial infarctions or demand ischemia, and hypotension (dobutamine and milrinone).[8] As a result of these undesirable outcomes, research is being conducted to develop new inotropes without such complications.[18]

Omecamtiv Mecarbil

Omecamtiv mecarbil, also known as CK-1827452, is a cardiac myosin activator. It increases the rate of ATP turnover in actin-myosin crosslinking during cardiac muscle contraction. As a result, it leads to increased numbers of myosin molecules on actin filaments, which leads to a more prolonged contractile force. The cardiac contraction is also more efficient because it increases intracellular calcium, thus the heart's oxygen and energy demand remains the same while the contractile force improves. Omecamtiv mecarbil is selective for cardiac myocytes and does not affect myosin molecules found in other muscular beds. A phase II clinical trial was performed in 45 subjects using omecamtiv mecarbil. It was noted that the drug increased the left ventricular (LV) ejection fraction and improved stroke volume. Side effects were related to high plasma concentrations of the medication and included chest pain, tachycardia, and myocardial ischemia.[19]

Sarcoplasmic Reticulum Calcium Adenosine Triphosphatase Gene Therapy

The SR calcium-ATPase (SERCA2a) enzyme regulates calcium homeostasis in the cardiac myocyte. The reuptake of calcium into the SR regulates cardiac relaxation and the release of calcium determines contractility. It has been noted that this enzyme is downregulated in patients with heart failure, and increased expression of this enzyme leads to improved survival due to enhanced contractility and cardiac metabolism. The ultimate utility of this treatment will likely be limited even to advanced heart failure patients because it is delivered directly to the coronaries and requires intense screening of patients who may react to antibodies in the viral vector capsid. It is, however, currently in clinical trials.[20]

Istaroxime is a new intravenous medication currently being studied. It actually stimulates SERCA2a expression and inhibits the action of the sodium-potassium ATPase. As a result, it enhances contractility by increasing intracellular calcium levels but it also enhances lusitropy by increasing the sequestration of calcium ions during diastole. This dual mechanism of action gives it the very unique properties of decreasing pulmonary capillary wedge pressure, decreasing heart rate, and increasing SBP, which is a combination of effects that no other inotropic agent can recreate.[21,22]

Levosimendan: A Calcium Sensitizer

Calcium sensitizers are a relatively new category of inotropes that enhance myocardial performance by increasing the affinity of TN-C to calcium. Levosimendan is a typical calcium sensitizer and potassium (K)-ATP channel opener that has emerged as an alternative option for inotropic support in patients with decompensated heart failure. The prolonged, enhanced contractility during systole (half-life of 80 hours) does not impair ventricular relaxation and it is not cleared by the kidneys. Also, levosimendan does not increase epinephrine or norepinephrine concentrations, thus avoiding resultant vasoconstriction, remodeling, or downregulation of cardiac receptor sensitivity. Levosimendan also acts on the K-ATP channels in smooth muscle, causing vasodilation. Thus, it acts as an effective afterload-reducing agent that also helps to increase cardiac output in the failing heart. Its vasodilatory effect varies according to the patient; however it is generally less than what is seen with milrinone.

Studies found that the use of levosimendan in severe heart failure was more favorable than conventional inotropic agents and it is currently approved for use in acutely decompensated heart failure in patients with low cardiac output in Europe (clinical trials in the United States are being conducted currently). For the cardiac anesthesiologist, levosimendan is mainly used in CABG surgery in patients with low ejection fraction. The medication is started after induction but before incision, and has been shown to increase LV contractility and reduce LV afterload effectively when continued in the postoperative period.[23]

Inhaled Agents

Advances in cardiovascular anesthesia have not just been in intravenous cardiovascular medications but also in the use of inhaled agents for the treatment of pulmonary hypertension and right heart failure. The main uses of inhaled agents are for left ventricular assist device placements, heart transplants and for patients with existing right heart failure or pulmonary hypertension undergoing cardiac or noncardiac surgery. These agents are beneficial in lowering pulmonary pressures in patients with reversible pulmonary hypertension, decreasing the afterload on the right heart, and increasing cardiac output.

The main benefit of the following inhaled agents is that the vasodilatory effects are limited to the pulmonary circulation and systemic hypotension is not seen as compared with intravenous administration. In addition, intravenous vasodilators will cause widespread vasodilation in the lungs, thus leading to intrapulmonary shunting where nonventilated areas of the lung receive perfusion. With inhaled agents, this is also avoided because their effect is only exerted on the alveolar-capillary membranes in ventilated portions of the lungs.

Nitric Oxide

The mainstay of therapy for pulmonary hypertension is the agent inhaled NO (iNO). NO is a relatively recent advancement in that it was discovered as an endogenous, endothelial-derived vasodilator in 1987 and was suggested for use in patients in 1991. It is a colorless, odorless gas that is diluted with pure nitrogen and stored in the absence of oxygen, thus it requires storage in specific gas tanks. It exerts its effect by diffusing into the smooth muscle of the pulmonary blood vessels and activating guanylate cyclase. Most iNO is converted to nitrate and excreted in the kidneys. In addition to its pulmonary vasodilatory effects, iNO has been shown to cause bronchodilation, and to act as an anti-inflammatory and anti-proliferative agent, thus mediating some of the effects of ischemia-reperfusion injury. The effective dose of iNO is between 5 to 40 ppm.

Toxicity associated with iNO therapy is related to the formation of nitrogen dioxide and methemoglobinemia. Nitrogen dioxide toxicity has been shown to occur at concentration of 1.5 ppm or more and manifests as increased airway reactivity or pulmonary edema in more extreme circumstances. Methemoglobinemia occurs as a byproduct of the reaction between iNO and hemoglobin. Both nitrogen dioxide and methemoglobinemia toxicity are exceedingly rare when concentrations of less than

80 ppm of iNO are used. Despite its safety, use of iNO is limited at some institutions due to its high cost and difficulty in administration.[24]

Of note, inhaled nitroprusside and inhaled nitroglycerin have also been investigated as potential pulmonary vasodilators and work through a similar pathway as iNO.[25]

Epoprostenol

Prostacyclin is an endogenous prostaglandin that causes smooth muscle relaxation via a cAMP pathway. The first prostacyclin analog to receive FDA approval for the treatment of pulmonary hypertension was epoprostenol but iloprost and treprostinil are also now available for use. Prostacyclin derivatives are also known to have antiplatelet effects and to inhibit the proliferation of vascular smooth muscle cells. Of note, the antiplatelet effect has only been shown in vitro and has not been shown to be of clinical significance. Epoprostenol must be delivered continuously because it has a short half-life of 3 to 6 minutes. Iloprost is intermediate acting with a half-life of about 20 to 30 minutes, thus it can be administered intermittently but on a frequent basis (generally 6–9 times a day). Treprostinil is the most promising because it has a half-life of about 4 hours and can be administered via nebulizer 4 times a day.[25]

Inhaled epoprostenol has been shown to be as effective at lowering pulmonary artery pressures and increasing cardiac output as iNO. It also is relatively free of toxicity and is easy to administer. The formulation comes in liquid form and is connected to a jet nebulizer in the inspiratory limb of the ventilatory circuit. The dose is initiated at 0.05 mcg/kg/min and can be titrated down to 0.01 mcg/kg/min before discontinuing its use.

REFERENCES

1. Lloyd-Jones D, Adams R, Carnethon M, et al. Heart disease and stroke statistics— 2009 update: a report from the American Heart Association statistics committee and stroke statistics subcommittee. Circulation 2009;119(3):480–6.
2. Baggish AL, van Kimmenade RR, Pinto Y, et al. New York Heart Association class versus amino-terminal pro-B type natriuretic peptide for acute heart failure prognosis. Biomarkers 2010;15(4):307–14.
3. Kangawa K, Matsuo H. Purification and complete amino acid sequence of human atrial natriuretic polypeptide (alpha-hANP). Biochem Biophys Res Commun 1984; 118:131–9.
4. Bhardwaj A, Januzzi JL Jr. Natriuretic peptide-guided management of acutely destabilized heart failure: rationale and treatment algorithm. Crit Pathw Cardiol 2009;8(4):146–50.
5. Reichert S, Ignaszewski A. Molecular and physiological effects of nesiritide. Can J Cardiol 2008;24(Suppl B):15B–8B.
6. Elkayam U, Akhter MW, Singh H, et al. Comparison of effects on left ventricular filling pressure of intravenous nesiritide and high-dose nitroglycerin in patients with decompensated heart failure. Am J Cardiol 2004;93(2):237–40.
7. Cardiovascular Pharmacology: an update 737. Available at: http://en.wikipedia.org/wiki/Cardiac_muscle. Accessed April 10, 2010.
8. Abraham WT, Adams KF, Fonarow GC, et al. In-hospital mortality in patients with acute decompensated heart failure requiring intravenous vasoactive medications: an analysis from the Acute Decompensated Heart Failure National Registry (ADHERE). J Am Coll Cardiol 2005;46:57–64.
9. Fellahi JL, Parienti JJ, Hanouz JL, et al. Perioperative use of dobutamine in cardiac surgery and adverse cardiac outcome: propensity-adjusted analyses. Anesthesiology 2008;108(6):979–87.

10. Teerlink JR. A novel approach to improve cardiac performance: cardiac myosin activators. Heart Fail Rev 2009;14(4):289–98.
11. Teerlink JR. Medscape. Available at: http://www.medscape.com/viewarticle/547591. Accessed April 10, 2010.
12. Available at: http://en.wikipedia.org/wiki/Diastolic_dysfunction#Pathophysiology. Accessed April 10, 2010.
13. Zile MR, Brutsaert DL. Causal mechanisms and treatment new concepts in diastolic dysfunction and diastolic heart failure: part II. Circulation 2002;105:1503–8.
14. Kwak YL, Oh YJ, Bang SO, et al. Comparison of the effects of nicardipine and sodium nitroprusside for control of increased blood pressure after coronary artery bypass graft surgery. J Int Med Res 2004;32:342–50.
15. Kenyon KW. Clevidipine: an ultra short-acting calcium channel antagonist for acute hypertension. Ann Pharmacother 2009;43(7):1258–65.
16. Varon J, Peacock W, Garrison N, et al. Prolonged infusion of clevidipine results in safe and predictable blood pressure control in patients with acute severe hypertension. Paper presented at the Annual Meeting of the American College of Chest Physicians. Chicago, October 20–25, 2007.
17. Nguyen HM, Ma K, Pham DQ. Clevidipine for the treatment of severe hypertension in adults. Clin Ther 2010;32:11–2.
18. Francis GS, Bartos JA, Adatya S. Inotropes. J Am Coll Cardiol 2014;63(20): 2069–78.
19. Cleland JG, Teerlink JR, Senior R, et al. The effects of the cardiac myosin activator, omecamtiv mecarbil, on cardiac function in systolic heart failure: a double-blind, placebo-controlled, crossover, dose ranging phase 2 trial. Lancet 2011;378:676–83.
20. Sabbah HN, Imai M, Cowart D, et al. Hemodynamic properties of a new-generation positive luso-inotropic agent for the acute treatment of advanced heart failure. Am J Cardiol 2007;99:41A–6A.
21. Gheorghiade M, Blair JE, Filippatos GS, et al. Hemodynamic, echocardiographic, and neurohormonal effects of istaroxime, a novel intravenous inotropic and lusitropic agent: a randomized controlled trial in patients hospitalized with heart failure. J Am Coll Cardiol 2008;51:2276–85.
22. Jessup M, Greenberg B, Mancini D, et al. Calcium Upregulation by Percutaneous Administration of Gene Therapy in Cardiac Disease (CUPID): a phase 2 trial of intracoronary gene therapy of sarcoplasmic reticulum Ca2þ-ATPase in patients with advanced heart failure. Circulation 2011;124:304–13.
23. Farmakis D, Alvarez J, Ben Gal T, et al. Levosimendan beyond inotropy and acute heart failure: Evidence of pleiotropic effects on the heart and other organs: an expert panel position paper. Int J Cardiol 2016;222:303–12.
24. Khan TA, Schnickel G, Ross D, et al. A prospective, randomized, crossover pilot study of inhaled nitric oxide versus inhaled prostacyclin in heart transplant and lung transplant recipients. J Thorac Cardiovasc Surg 2009;138:1417–24.
25. Thunberg VA, Morozowich ST, Ramakrishna H. Inhaled therapy for the management of perioperative pulmonary hypertension. Ann Card Anaesth 2015;18(3): 394–402.

Pharmacogenomics in Anesthesia

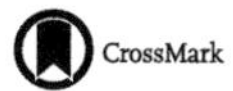

Ramsey Saba, MD[a], Alan D. Kaye, MD, PhD, DABA, DABPM, DABIPP[b], Richard D. Urman, MD, MBA[a,*]

KEYWORDS

- Allele • Homozygous • Heterozygous • Genotype • Phenotype
- Pharmacogenomics • Polymorphisms • Single-nucleotide polymorphisms (SNP)
- Genetics

KEY POINTS

- There are a growing number of genomic variations that alter the standard expected course of neuromuscular blocking agents.
- Three common points of genomic expression that lead to opioid interpatient variability include opioid transportation, receptor molecules, and enzymes involved in opioid metabolism.
- There is growing evidence characterizing pharmacogenomics interactions associated with malignant hyperthermia and postoperative nausea and vomiting.
- Better understanding of genetic predisposition to bleeding and arrhythmias following cardiac surgery may change management recommendations.

INTRODUCTION

Much of clinicians' daily practice involves the science of drugs and how to tailor them to each individual patient. It is well documented that different drugs can have much interpatient variability related to various environmental factors, including diet, social habits, and geographic influence. Clinicians are now looking more into the intrinsic causes of variability; notably, differences in a patient's genome. A better understanding of genomic influences on anesthesia may allow a more individually tailored anesthetic and ultimately lead to better outcomes, decreased hospital stays, and improved patient satisfaction. In this article we review several studies and discuss the current role of genetics in drug response-specifically within the realm of anesthesia.

Disclosure Statement: The authors have nothing to disclose.

[a] Department of Anesthesiology, Perioperative and Pain Medicine, Brigham and Women's Hospital, Harvard Medical School, 75 Francis Street, Boston, MA 02115, USA; [b] Department of Anesthesiology and Pain Medicine, LSU Health Science Center, Louisiana State University School of Medicine, 1542 Tulane Avenue, Room 659, New Orleans, LA 70112, USA
* Corresponding author.
E-mail address: urmanr@gmail.com

Anesthesiology Clin 35 (2017) 285–294
http://dx.doi.org/10.1016/j.anclin.2017.01.014 anesthesiology.theclinics.com
1932-2275/17/

The concept of pharmacogenetics was first described by geneticist Friedrich Vogel[1] in the late 1950s. He described polymorphisms in the acetylation of isoniazid. This antituberculosis drug is metabolized by acetylation in the liver. Some individuals were slow inactivators of the drug and some were faster. As one would expect, failure rates were higher for fast-activators and slow-inactivators had a higher incidence of toxicity.[2] In this example, the study of inherited differences in drug metabolism is referred to as pharmacogenetics. In a much broader sense, pharmacogenomics refers to the many different genes that determine drug behavior. It is a description of how chromosomal variations affect pharmacologic responses.[3] Much of this translates to polymorphisms that cause variations in drug transporters, metabolizing enzymes, and receptors.[4]

NEUROMUSCULAR BLOCKING AGENTS

In 1957, Kalow and Gunn[5] described an inherited variation in drug metabolism involving succinylcholine and serum cholinesterases. Broad differences in duration of apnea due to succinylcholine administration (as now generally understood by most anesthesiologists) is secondary to well-described polymorphisms in metabolism.

The level and quality of plasma cholinesterase activity (pseudocholinesterase, butyrylcholinesterase [BCHE]) is now understood to determine the clinical effects of several pharmacologic agents. Of the neuromuscular blocking agents, succinylcholine and mivacurium are well-described to be metabolized by these cholinesterases.[6]

Currently, all inherited causes of clinically relevant BCHE deficiency are secondary to point mutations located on chromosome 3.[7] Genetic variations in the BChE have expanded from only 4 known forms to more than 20 identifiable variants in the last several years. This has greatly increased the complexity of diagnosis and interpretation of these genetic traits.[4] More than 96% of the population is homozygous for the normal pseudocholinesterase genotype (U, representing the usual variant) with 3% to 4% heterozygous for the atypical genes. It is estimated that 1 in 2800 people are homozygous for the autosomal-recessive genes of an atypical enzyme.[8,9]

The 2 most common mutations are the A-variant (atypical, or dibucaine resistant; Asp70Gly) and the K-variant (Ala539Thr), which are both common among whites.[10,11] Those who are heterozygous for the K- or A-variant can have prolonged muscle relaxation for up to an hour (3–8 times longer) after 1 to 1.5 mg/kg administration of succinylcholine. Homozygous expression of these alleles can prolong neuromuscular block for up to 60 times longer compared with the normal allele.[3] One of the most serious and rare variants is known as the S-variant. A person homozygous for the S genotype will have no pseudocholinesterase activity and may experience paralysis for up to 8 hours with a single induction dose of succinylcholine.[12,13] Other well-described variants include the fluoride-resistant (F)-variant (with altered hydrolyzing activity) and 2 quantitative variants with decreased enzyme concentration (H, J) (**Table 1**).

Unlike succinylcholine, mivacurium is a benzylisoquinolinium nondepolarizing neuromuscular blocker that has an onset of action of 2 to 3 minutes and a duration of action of 12 to 20 minutes. This duration of action is approximately twice that of succinylcholine and less than half of intermediate-acting nondepolarizing neuromuscular blockers.[13] Because it is also metabolized by pseudocholinesterase, it is not surprising that longer durations of action are seen in many of the described variants. When used for neuromuscular blockade, mivacurium is found to be 4 to 5 times more potent in patients homozygous for atypical or silent genes compared with normal plasma cholinesterase.[14] Of note, mivacurium is currently not being marketed in the United States.

Table 1
Variants of butyrylcholinesterase with activity of succinylcholine (~1–1.5 mg/kg)

Name	Abbreviation	Mutation	Allele Frequency (General Population)	Description	Estimated Paralysis
Usual	U	—	98%	Normal	~5 min
Atypical	A	A209 G	Homozygote: .03%-.01%, Heterozygote: 4%	Reduced activity, dibucaine-resistant	>2 h
Fluoride-resistant	F	C728 T, G1169 T	Homozygote: .0007%	Reduced activity, fluoride-resistant	1–2 h
Silent	S	Multiple	Homozygote: .01%-.008%	No activity	3–4+h
H	H	G424 A	?	Approximately 10% reduced concentration	?
J	J	A1490 T	?	Approximately 33% reduced concentration	?
K	K	G1615 A	Homozygote: 1.5%	Approximately 66% reduced concentration	<1 h

Adapted from Levano S, Ginz H, Siegemund M, et al. Genotyping the butyrylcholinesterase in patients with prolonged neuromuscular block after succinylcholine. Anesthesiology 2005;102(3):532; and Soliday FK, Conley YP, Henker R. Pseudocholinesterase deficiency: a comprehensive review of genetic, acquired, and drug influences. AANA J 2010;78(4):315.

OPIOIDS

There are many factors that determine opioid responses in individuals. Some of these include variations in an individuals' metabolism, receptors, and transporter proteins.

Metabolism

Many variations of cytochrome enzymes between individuals can determine what effect opioid metabolism will have on an individual. Codeine, for example, is metabolized into its active metabolite (morphine) by CYP2D6.[15] Patients with increased CYP2D6 metabolism (often referred to as ultrarapid metabolizers) can have high levels of morphine with standard dosing. Similarly, tramadol and hydrocodone are also metabolized by CYP2D6 with ultrarapid metabolizers at a higher risk of experiencing life-threatening side effects,[16,17] whereas poor metabolizers may be mostly free of any adverse reactions.

Similarly, fentanyl has been shown to be metabolized in part by CYP3A4. One study examined the effects of CYP3A4 polymorphisms on transdermal fentanyl metabolism.[18] It was shown that fentanyl absorption rates were higher in the CYP3A5*3/*3 group than in the *1/*1 and *1/*3 groups and led to a greater incidence of central adverse events.

Catechol-O-methyltransferase (COMT) is involved in metabolism of catecholamines and is widely associated with neurotransmission. It is estimated that 10% of variability in all pain sensitivity is associated with single nucleotide polymorphisms in COMT.[19]

One study examined whether the COMT gene was useful in predicting morphine requirements. It found that carriers of COMT Val/Val and Val/Met genotypes required

63% and 23%, respectively, higher doses of morphine compared with the Met/Met genotype.[20]

Receptors

There are several receptors involved with opioid analgesia. The 3 most well-known are mu, kappa, and delta receptors, which are coded for by the OPRM1, OPRK1, and OPRD1 genes, respectively.[19] Each receptor has been identified in playing various roles in opioid clinical effects. The mu-opioid receptor, for instance has been identified as the primary analgesic responding receptor to opioids.[21] The kappa-opioid receptor has been shown to produce aversive states and is helpful in preventing opioid reinforcement. The delta-receptor, similarly, has shown some involvement in opioid dependence.[22]

There is some evidence that the OPRM1 GG genotype requires 93% higher morphine dose compared with the AA genotype.[20] Regarding commonly used opioids (nalbuphine, pentazocine, and butorphanol) using OPRK1, there is some evidence to suggest gender differences in response to opioids.[23]

Transporters

One of the better understood opioid transporters is the P-glycoprotein transporter (encoded by ABCB1) found along the blood-brain barrier.[24] Polymorphisms in this transporter have been shown to effect opioid variability on respiratory depression. Children with GG and GA genotypes of ABCB1 polymorphism (rs9282564) were shown to have higher risk of respiratory depression and prolonged hospital stay.[24]

Mutations in ABCB1 have also been associated with higher methadone doses in methadone-maintained heroin addicts.[19]

LOCAL ANESTHETICS

Local anesthetics primarily work on sodium channels and have varying methods of metabolism. Amides, including lidocaine and bupivacaine, are metabolized by CYP3A4 and ropivacaine by CYP1A2.[25] One study investigated mutations in the Nav1.7-N395 K channel and its effect on lidocaine.[26] The N395 K mutation significantly reduced use-dependent inhibition of lidocaine on both resting and inactivated Nav1.7.

Notably, MC1R-variants (in a study examining women with red hair) were found to be more resistant to the effects of subcutaneous lidocaine.[27]

INHALATION ANESTHETICS

The most important route for elimination of inhalation anesthetics is the alveolus. There is partial elimination through biotransformation (through CYP2E1) but this plays a minimal role in anesthetic elimination. Inhalation anesthetics that undergo more extensive metabolism (eg, methoxyflurane) are more affected by changes in enzymatic biotransformation.[28] Twenty percent to 50% of halothane, 2% of sevoflurane, less than 1% of isoflurane, and 0.1% of desflurane are metabolized by enzymes.[25] Halothane is more soluble than sevoflurane yet has a faster elimination due to its greater biotransformation through CYP2E1.[28] Although genetic variations in CYP2E1 could account for small differences in elimination, the largest contributor to is through exhalation, decreasing the clinical relevance of these variations in commonly used inhalation anesthetics.

Sevoflurane is known to exert effects on gamma-aminobutyric acid (GABA)ergic transmission.[29] One Korean study investigated the effects of polymorphisms in

GABR[gamma]2 toward emergence agitation in the pediatric population. The study suggests that those with the AA genotype of GABR[gamma]2 at position 3145 in intron A/G had an increased incidence of emergence agitation compared with the non-AA group.[29]

Melanocortin-1 receptor (MC1R) mutations have long been associated with an increased desflurane anesthetic requirement.[25 30] Interestingly, the phenotype of all red haired individuals can be traced to distinct mutations of the MC1R gene on chromosome 16.[30] This association may explain why red hair seems to be a distinct phenotype that can be traced to specific mutations in a well-described gene. Compared with women with dark hair, women with red hair require almost 20% more desflurane to achieve the same effect and are also notably more resistant to the effects of subcutaneous lidocaine (see previous discussion).[27]

MALIGNANT HYPERTHERMIA

The underlying effect of 1 of the triggers of malignant hyperthermia (MH) is the rapid lease of calcium from the sarcoplasmic reticulum. This trigger often results in a hypermetabolic state that, if left untreated, can lead to cardiovascular collapse and even death. There is much observation support that a single RYR1 mutation is the cause of MH in pig studies, as well as some human families.[31] The specific mutation is a substitution of Cys for Arg614. This mutation, however, is not seen in all human families with MH. To date, there are more than 90 different mutations that have been associated with the RYR-1 gene mutation on chromosome 19q13.1 and 25 of these mutations are causal for MH (of note, there are at least 6 genetic loci other than RYR1 that have been implicated in MH but are not causal).[32] There are several inherited disorders that are associated with MH.[33] Central core disease (CCD) is a mainly autosomal dominant inherited disease characterized by muscle weakness (muscles showing a predominance of type 1 fibers). One study shows that more than 93% of Japanese CCD patients exhibit an RYR1-variant.[34] Other MH susceptible myopathies include myotonic muscular dystrophy (recessive inheritance), centronuclear myopathy, and King-Denborough syndrome.[33]

BENZODIAZEPINES

Most benzodiazepines are metabolized by hepatic CYP enzymes. Polymorphisms and induced variations in CYP enzymes have been shown to effect drug metabolism and, therefore, their effects. The CYP3A4/5 enzymes, for instance, are primarily responsible for the metabolism of midazolam. Those homozygous for CYP3A5*3 were found to have a greater than 50% induction of these enzymes.[25] Despite these differences, the clinical significance of these polymorphisms is relatively small.[3] There is also much conflicting evidence regarding variations in midazolam clearance when comparing different polymorphisms (CYP3A5*1/*3 and CYP3A5*3/*3).[35] Although midazolam remains the most extensively used benzodiazepine premedication for operations, evidence regarding clinical variations in polymorphisms of CYP3A5 remains inconclusive. Diazepam is metabolized to nordiazepam via CYP3A4 and CYP2C19 ant to temazepam (active) via CYP3A4. Nordiazepam is then metabolized to oxazepam (active) via CYP3A4. Increases in plasma levels of diazepam have been noted in m1-variants of the CYP2C19 enzymes and even higher levels in m1 homozygous individuals.[36] Notably, the half-life of diazepam in individuals homozygous for the A-allele of the cytochrome CYP2C19 G681 A polymorphism is 4 times longer than those homozygous for the G-allele. Clinically, these variations may manifest as prolonged sedation (**Table 2**).[3]

Table 2
CYP enzymes involved in benzodiazepine metabolism

Benzodiazepines	CYP Enzymes Studied In Vivo
Alprazolam	CYP3A4/5
Brotizolam	3A4
Clobazam	2C19, 3A4
Diazepam	2C19, 3A4
Etizolam	2C19, 3A4
Flunitrazepam	2C19, 3A4
Midazolam	3A4/5
Quazepam	2C19, 3A4
Triazolam	3A4

Data from Fukasawa T, Suzuki A, Otani K. Effects of genetic polymorphism of cytochrome P450 enzymes on the pharmacokinetics of benzodiazepines. J Clin Pharm Ther 2007;32(4):336.

POSTOPERATIVE NAUSEA AND VOMITING

It has been shown that 5-hydroxytryptamine type 3 (5-HT3) antagonism can significantly reduce postoperative nausea and vomiting (PONV), although 35% of patients treated with ondansetron will still experience PONV.[37] One study investigates whether Y129s and −100_-102AAG deletion polymorphisms (5-HT3B, receptor gene deletion polymorphisms) affect the efficacy of ondansetron.[37] It showed a significant association between the −100_-1-2AAG deletion polymorphism and the efficacy of ondansetron with a higher incidence of PONV in homomutant genotypes.[37]

SNPs for dopamine type 2 receptors have also been shown to be related to PONV. One study involving 1070 subjects showed that those with the DRD2 Taq IA polymorphism had a higher incidence of early PONV.[38]

There are also several mu-opioid and COMT gene polymorphisms that affect morphine analgesia. This translates to variations in opioid-related side effects in the postoperative period. One study shows that heterozygous patients with mu-opioid receptor A118 G and COMT G1947 A mutation consumed less morphine in the postanesthetic recovery room and, as a likely effect, had nausea scores that were significantly lower compared with homozygous patients (**Table 3**).[39,40]

CARDIOVASCULAR GENOMICS

There is emerging evidence that patients' genetic makeup may predispose them to adverse outcomes following cardiac surgery. One cardiac surgery review discusses the role of various genetic polymorphisms in determining adverse outcomes, such as perioperative bleeding, myocardial injury or infarction, and atrial fibrillation (AF).[40] It concludes that the overall genetic effect on outcome is typically the sum of numerous small genetic effects modified by nongenetic factors. There remains considerable interindividual variability in both incidence and severity of adverse outcomes following cardiac surgery. With growing genomic correlations, however, clinically significant management recommendations may be on the horizon.

Coagulation Variability

There are several well-known inherited coagulation deficiencies that have been consistently shown to correlate with increased propensity for bleeding. Of these

Table 3
Candidate genes that affect postoperative nausea and vomiting

Gene (Molecule)	Function
HTR3A (5-hydroxytryptamine type 3 receptor subunit A)	Neural Signaling
HTR3B (5-hydroxytryptamine type 3 receptor subunit B)	Neural Signaling
OPRM1 (opioid receptor, mu 1)	Neural Signaling
CHRM3 (Muscarinic acetylcholine receptor 3 subtype)	Neural Signaling
DRD2 (Dopamine type 2 receptor)	Neural Signaling
COMT (Catechol-o-methyl transferase)	Degradation of catecholamines
ABCB1 (Adenosine triphosphate-binding cassette subfamily B member 1)	Blood-brain barrier transporter
CYP2D6 (cytochrome P450 superfamily enzyme)	Drug metabolism

Adapted from Horn CC, Wallisch WJ, Homanics GE, et al. Pathophysiological and neurochemical mechanisms of postoperative nausea and vomiting. Eur J Pharmacol 2014;722: 55–66; with permission.

inherited deficiencies, von Willebrand disease, together with the well-established X-linked inherited diseases hemophilia A and B make up 95% to 97% of deficiencies in coagulation factors.[41] These inherited deficiencies are well correlated with intraoperative propensity to bleed. Patients with these known deficiencies often present during childhood or early genetic testing, given familial inheritance patterns. When presenting for surgery, their known bleeding risk allows for perioperative changes in clinical management (ie, administration of factor concentrate or synthetic analogues such as desmopressin and further transfusion preparations).

Thrombotic outcomes after cardiac surgery (stroke, pulmonary embolism, and coronary graft thrombosis) play another key role at the other end of the spectrum.

One review describes several genetic polymorphisms in the hemostatic system, with multiple suggestive and established associations of their phenotype with disease. Polymorphisms in *Fibrinogen β-chain −455 G/A*, *Fibrinogen β-chain −854 G/A*, and *Fibrinogen β-chain Bcl1*, for example, have all been associated with elevated plasma fibrinogen levels. This phenotypic elevation has consistently been shown to be associated with arterial thrombotic disease, identifying itself as an independent relative risk factor for ischemic stroke, myocardial infarction, and peripheral vascular disease.[42] Despite this correlation, there is still no recommendation for screening due to the lack of evidence to indicate any prognostic or therapeutic consequence within the general population.[43]

There are, however, several prothrombotic genotypes associated with risk of coronary graft thrombosis and myocardial injury after surgery that have well-established clinical consequences. One of these is a prothrombotic point mutation in coagulation factor V (factor V Leiden [FVL]). This resulting protein C resistance has been consistently shown to increase the risk of myocardial infarction. One population-based case-control study showed an increased risk of myocardial infarction up to 50% (compared with 1.8% and 1.2% in heterozygous and control subjects, respectively).[44]

Atrial Fibrillation

In an analysis of 8 large cardiac surgery trials totaling 20,193 subjects, the incidence of postoperative AF (PoAF) was estimated to be 26% and ranged from 17% to 35%, typically occurring after the second or third postoperative day.[45,46] One study determined that AF itself can independently prolong hospital stay after coronary artery bypass surgery.[47] This implicates that successful treatment and prevention of AF could contribute to major reductions in consumption of health care resources in patients with CABG.

One study evaluated polymorphisms in 3 genes (IL-6, ACE, and ApOE), which have been previously implicated in PoAF, and how they correlate with the disease. They found that a single locus effect of IL-6 could correctly predict disease status with 58.8% accuracy. Furthermore, there exists an interaction between history AF and length of hospital stay that can predict disease status with 68.34% accuracy.[48]

As this disease is increasingly predicted, further potentially preventative action can be taken. One analysis of a large multicenter international cohort suggests that treatment with beta-blockers, angiotensin converting enzyme (ACE) inhibitors, and/or nonsteroidal anti-inflammatory drugs may offer protection from after CABG surgery.[49] Other implications from the study include decreased AF infection, renal, and neurologic complications after CABG from decreasing recurrent AF episodes, as well as, ultimately, decreasing hospital stays.

One study has shown associations between renin-angiotensin system (RAS) gene polymorphism and nonfamilial structural AF.[50] Significant associations were specifically found in single-locus analysis of ACE gene insertion or deletion polymorphisms (*M235 T*, G-*6A*, and *G-217A*). These data may suggest a correlation with the known use of ACE-I therapy in cardiac surgery in reducing the incidence of PoAF.[49] Despite this observation, there has yet to be shown a direct correlation of genetic variants in the RAS with the incidence of PoAF.

SUMMARY

Although a relatively young field, pharmacogenomics has already shown that a better understanding of a person's particular genome can cater to individualized care. Despite the vast amount of research on these well-described anesthetic diseases (MH, pseudocholinesterase deficiency, PONV) the research is just beginning to describe the various polymorphisms that contribute to them. A better understanding of these susceptible genomes will lead to better consideration of drug choices. This will ultimately decrease the incidence of adverse events and hospital stays, as well as increase patient satisfaction.

REFERENCES

1. Vogel F. Moderne probleme der humangenetik. Ergeb Inn Med Kinderheilkd 1959;12:52–125 [in German].
2. Davidson RG. PDQ medical genetics. Hamilton (Ontario): BC Decker; 2002.
3. Palmer SN, Giesecke NM, Simon CB, et al. Pharmacogenetics of anesthetic and analgesic agents. Anesthesiology 2005;102(3):663–71.
4. Iohom G. Principles of pharmacogenetics–implications for the anaesthetist. Br J Anaesth 2004;93(3):440–50.
5. Kalow W, Gunn DR. Apnea. Anesthesiol 1958;19(1):125.
6. Jensen FS, Schwartz M, Viby-Mogensen J. Identification of human plasma cholinesterase variants using molecular biological techniques. Acta Anaesthesiol Scand 1995;39(2):142–9.
7. Faust RJ. Prolongation of succinylcholine effect. In: Faust RJ, editor. Anesthesiology review. New York: Churchill Livingstone; 2002. p. 137–8.
8. Chung SJ, August AD. Prolonged postoperative succinylcholine-induced apnea with pseudocholinesterase deficiency. J Tenn Med Assoc 1982;75(8):535–6.

9. Stoelting RK, Dierdorf SF. Anesthesia and CoExisting diseases. New York: Churchill Livingstone Inc; 1983. p. 329.
10. Galley HF, Mahdy A, Lowes DA. Pharmacogenetics and anesthesiologists. Pharmacogenomics 2005;6(8):849–56.
11. Gätke MR, Viby-Mogensen J, Bundgaard JR. Rapid simultaneous genotyping of the frequent butyrylcholinesterase variants Asp70Gly and Ala539Thr with fluorescent hybridization probes. Scand J Clin Lab Invest 2002;62(5):375–83.
12. Ama T, Bounmythavong S, Blaze J, et al. Implications of pharmacogenomics for anesthesia providers. AANA J 2010;78(5):393–9.
13. Miller RD, Pardo M, Stoelting RK. Basics of anesthesia. Philadelphia: Elsevier Health Sciences; 2011.
14. Ostergaard D, Jensen FS, Theil Skovgaard L, et al. Dose-response relationship for mivacurium inpatients with phenotypically abnormal plasma cholinesterase activity. Acta Anaesthesiol Scand 1995;39(8):1016–8.
15. Linares OA, Fudin J, Schiesser WE, et al. CYP2D6 phenotype-specific codeine population pharmacokinetics. J Pain Palliat Care Pharmacother 2015;29(1):4–15.
16. Kapur BM, Prateek KL, Julie LV. Pharmacogenetics of chronic pain management. Clin Biochem 2014;47(13–14):1169–87.
17. Lassen D, Per D, Brøsen K. The pharmacogenetics of tramadol. Clin Pharmacokinet 2015;54(8):825–36.
18. Takashina Y, Naito T, Mino Y, et al. Impact of CYP3A5 and ABCB1 gene polymorphisms on fentanyl pharmacokinetics and clinical responses in cancer patients undergoing conversion to a transdermal system. Drug Metab Pharmacokinet 2012;27(4):414–21.
19. Trescot AM, Faynboym S. A review of the role of genetic testing in pain medicine. Pain Physician 2014;17:425–45.
20. Reyes-Gibby CC, Shete S, Rakvåg T, et al. Exploring joint effects of genes and the clinical efficacy of morphine for cancer pain: OPRM1 and COMT Gene. Pain 2007;130(1):25–30.
21. Cregg R, Russo G, Gubbay A, et al. Pharmacogenetics of analgesic drugs. Br J Pain 2013;7(4):189–208.
22. Zhang H, Gelernter J, Gruen JR, et al. Functional impact of a single-nucleotide polymorphism in the OPRD1 promoter region. J Hum Genet 2010;55(5):278–84.
23. Gear RW, Gordon NC, Hossaini-Zadeh M, et al. A subanalgesic dose of morphine eliminates nalbuphine anti-analgesia in postoperative pain. J Pain 2008;9(4): 337–41.
24. Sadhasivam S, Chidambaran V, Zhang X, et al. Opioid-induced respiratory depression: ABCB1 transporter pharmacogenetics. Pharmacogenomics J 2014;15(2): 119–26.
25. Cohen M, Sadhasivam S, Vinks AA. Pharmacogenetics in perioperative medicine. Curr Opin Anaesthesiol 2012;25(4):419–27.
26. Sheets PL, Jackson JO, Waxman SG, et al. A Na v. 1.7 channel mutation associated with hereditary erythromelalgia contributes to neuronal hyperexcitability and displays reduced lidocaine sensitivity. J Physiol 2007;581(3):1019–31.
27. Bentov I. Anesthetic implications of pharmacogenetics. ASA Refresher Courses in Anesthesiology 2014;42(1):18–22.
28. Morgan GE, Maged SM, Murray MJ. Clinical anesthesiology. New York: Lange Medical/McGraw Hill Medical Pub Division; 2006.
29. Park CS, Shin C, Jin Park H, et al. The influence of GABA A $\gamma 2$ genetic polymorphism on the emergence agitation induced by sevoflurane. Korean J Anesthesiol 2008;55(2):139.

30. Liem EB, Lin CM, Suleman MI, et al. Anesthetic requirement is increased in redheads. Anesthesiology 2004;101(2):279–83.
31. Maclennan DH. The genetic basis of malignant hyperthermia. Trends Pharmacol Sci 1992;13:330–4.
32. Rosenberg H, Davis M, James D, et al. Malignant hyperthermia. Orphanet J Rare Dis 2007;2(1):21.
33. Rosenberg H, Pollock N, Schiemann A, et al. Malignant hyperthermia: a review. Orphanet J Rare Dis 2015;10(1):93.
34. Wu S. Central core disease is due to RYR1 mutations in more than 90% of patients. Brain 2006;129(6):1470–80.
35. Fukasawa T, Suzuki A, Otani K. Effects of genetic polymorphism of cytochrome p450 enzymes on the pharmacokinetics of benzodiazepines. J Clin Pharm Ther 2007;32(4):333–41.
36. Trescot AM. Genetics and implications in perioperative analgesia. Best Pract Res Clin Anaesthesiol 2014;28(2):153–66.
37. Kim MS, Lee JR, Choi EM, et al. Association of 5-HT3B receptor gene polymorphisms with the efficacy of ondansetron for postoperative nausea and vomiting. Yonsei Med J 2015;56(5):1415.
38. Nakagawa M, Kuri M, Kambara N, et al. Dopamine D2 receptor taq ia polymorphism is associated with postoperative nausea and vomiting. J Anesth 2008; 22(4):397–403.
39. Kolesnikov Y, Gabovits B, Levin A, et al. Combined Catechol-O-Methyltransferase and μ-Opioid receptor gene polymorphisms affect morphine postoperative analgesia and central side effects. Anesth Analg 2011;112(2):448–53.
40. Perry TE, Muehlschlegel JD, Body SC. Genomics: risk and outcomes in cardiac surgery. Anesthesiol Clin 2008;26(3):399–417.
41. Peyvandi F, Jayandharan G, Chandy M, et al. Genetic diagnosis of haemophilia and other inherited bleeding disorders. Haemophilia 2006;12(S3):82–9.
42. Voetsch B, Loscalzo J. Genetic determinants of arterial thrombosis. Arterioscler Thromb Vasc Biol 2003;24(2):216–29.
43. Reiner AP, Siscovick DS, Rosendaal FR. Hemostatic risk factors and arterial thrombotic disease. Thromb Haemost 2001;85:584–95.
44. Doggen CJ, Cats VM, Bertina RM, et al. Interaction of coagulation defects and cardiovascular risk factors: increased risk of myocardial infarction associated with factor V Leiden or Prothrombin 20210A. Circulation 1998;97(11):1037–41.
45. Didomenico RJ, Massad MG. Pharmacologic strategies for prevention of atrial fibrillation after open heart surgery. Ann Thorac Surg 2005;79(2):728–40.
46. Maisel WH. Atrial fibrillation after cardiac surgery. Ann Intern Med 2001;135(12): 1061.
47. Tamis JE, Steinberg JS. Atrial fibrillation independently prolongs hospital stay after coronary artery bypass surgery. Clin Cardiol 2000;23(3):155–9.
48. Motsinger AA, Donahue BS, Brown NJ, et al. Risk factor interactions and genetic effects associated with post-operative atrial fibrillation. Pac Symp Biocomput 2006;584–95.
49. Mathew JP. A multicenter risk index for atrial fibrillation after cardiac surgery. JAMA 2004;291(14):1720.
50. Tsai CT. Renin-angiotensin system gene polymorphisms and atrial fibrillation. Circulation 2004;109(13):1640–6.

Pharmacogenomics in Pain Management

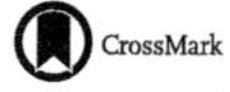

Ramsey Saba, MD[a], Alan D. Kaye, MD, PhD, DABA, DABPM, DABIPP[b],
Richard D. Urman, MD, MBA[a,*]

KEYWORDS

- Allele • Haplotype • Homozygous • Heterozygous • Genotype
- Pharmacogenomics • Polymorphisms • Single-nucleotide polymorphisms (SNP)
- Pain

KEY POINTS

- Opioid classes have a wide variability in clinical manifestations that can partly be explained by differences in metabolism and receptor molecules.
- There are several cytochrome enzymes involved in ketamine metabolism but strong genetic correlations between metabolism variations and clinical manifestation have yet to be identified.
- Catechol-O-methyltransferase plays an important role in variability of pain sensitivity, and certain alleles may predispose patients to higher opioid requirements for pain control.
- Pharmacogenomics nonsteroidal anti-inflammatory drugs are increasingly better understood and, in some instances, have already led to changes in dosing recommendations.

INTRODUCTION

Pharmacogenomics is a relatively new field that combines pharmacology and genomics to develop effective, safe medications and dosages.[1] This allows for pharmacologic tailoring of treatment to individuals. Much of this field can be applicable to understanding pain management and various responses to drugs seen in the clinical setting. This inter-individual variability is still under review and a better understanding of pharmacogenomics is key to improving patient care.

Pain management is often very costly and time consuming. It is estimated that more than $600 billion is spent annually on managing chronic pain.[2] Some of this cost is attributed to adverse outcomes and lengthened hospital stays. With pharmacogenomics there is potential to improve pain management by predicting outcomes before

Disclosure Statement: The authors have nothing to disclose.
[a] Department of Anesthesiology, Perioperative and Pain Medicine, Harvard Medical School, Brigham and Women's Hospital, 75 Francis Street, Boston, MA 02115, USA; [b] Department of Anesthesiology and Pain Medicine, Louisiana State University School of Medicine, LSU Health Science Center, 1542 Tulane Avenue, Room 659, New Orleans, LA 70112, USA
* Corresponding author.
E-mail address: urmanr@gmail.com

Anesthesiology Clin 35 (2017) 295–304
http://dx.doi.org/10.1016/j.anclin.2017.01.015 **anesthesiology.theclinics.com**
1932-2275/17/

before the medication is even prescribed. According to the US Food and Drug (FDA) administration there are more than 2 million serious adverse drug reactions yearly, with 100,000 resulting in death. Adverse drug reactions are estimated to cost $136 billion annually and are known to increase average length of hospital stay and mortality.[3]

Noninvasive saliva testing, for instance, could someday allow clinicians to determine the most appropriate medication for an individual patient, decreasing the adverse effects and increasing efficacy.[4]

METABOLISM VARIABILITY

There are many enzymes that have been shown to be associated with the metabolism of opioids. This allows room for genetic variability to play a role in both the efficacy and toxicity of these drugs. This variability comes in several forms but can be broadly classified as extensive-metabolism, intermediate-metabolism, poor-metabolism, or ultra-metabolism.[5] An extensive metabolizer would have 2 normal alleles, an intermediate metabolizer would have 1 normal and 1 reduced allele, and a poor metabolizer would have 2 mutant alleles.

One example of opioid metabolism variability is seen when looking at polymorphisms in CYP2D6. Cytochrome enzymes are well-known to be involved in the metabolism of many drugs, including many opioids. There are at least 80 identified CYP2D6 alleles, which leaves much room for enzymatic variability, from 1% to 200% when compared with the wild-type allele.[6]

The CYP2D6 allele is also known to vary among ethnicities. This assembly of allele frequencies may require a larger study for more accurate assessment but also better correlation with clinical responses. The clinical responses may vary significantly as well, given that the nonfunctioning and reduced functioning alleles noted in **Table 1** also may vary in response on a functional gradient.[7]

WEAK OPIOIDS

Codeine

Codeine is considered a weak opioid and is widely used for its analgesic effects. Many practitioners are familiar with CYP2D6 polymorphisms and its effect on codeine metabolism. Plasma codeine and its active metabolites (eg, morphine) have varying pharmacokinetic pathways depending on patient CYP2D6 makeup.[8] Ultrametabolizers of codeine can have high levels of morphine after standard dosing, whereas patients who are poor metabolizers will experience minimal effects.

Table 1
Median frequency of CYP2D6 alleles classified as functional, nonfunctional, and reduced function based on different ethnicities

Ethnicity	Functional Allele (%)	Nonfunctional Allele (%)	Reduced Functioning Allele (%)
Whites	71	26	1–10
Asians	~50	1–10	~40
Africans	50–55	1–10	30–40
African Americans	~50	10–20	30–40

Adapted from Bradford LD. CYP2D6 Allele Frequency in European Caucasians, Asians, Africans and their descendants. Pharmacogenomics 2002;3(2):230.

One case report published in 2006 describes the death of a 13-day-old infant whose mother was prescribed codeine for episiotomy pain. The mother's breastmilk was found to have higher than expected levels of morphine. After further review, she was found to be an ultrametabolizer of codeine and the infant had died from opioid toxicity secondary to increased morphine levels in breastmilk.[9]

Another case report from 2004 describes a man in his 60s who was prescribed codeine for cough suppression. Shortly afterward he was found to deteriorate rapidly, which was ultimately found to be secondary to his ultrametabolism of codeine (due to 3 or more functional alleles). He was given naloxone with rapid improvement of his symptoms.[10]

Hydrocodone

Similar to codeine, hydrocodone is metabolized by CYP2D6 to its active metabolite hydromorphone. This metabolite has a high affinity for the mu receptor. One study examined 25,200 urine samples of subjects taking hydrocodone and found much variability in hydrocodone or hydromorphone variability.[11] They were able to show through urine testing that 0.6% of participators were ultrametabolizers and 4% were poor metabolizers of hydrocodone.

Another study examined 158 women scheduled for C-sections that received hydrocodone 24 hours after surgery for postoperative pain control.[12] On postoperative day 3, serum opioid concentrations were examined and correlated to their OPRM1 genotype (see later discussion). The study found an association between pain relief and total hydrocodone dose with subjects homozygous for 118A allele (AA) of the OPRM1 gene but not in patients with 118G allele (AG or GG).

Tramadol

Tramadol hydrochloride is another commonly used weak opioid analgesic. It is a synthetic codeine analogue that inhibits the reuptake of serotonin and norepinephrine.[13] Similar to codeine and hydrocodone, one of its metabolizers is CYP2D6. Other genetic variations that determine the pharmacokinetics and/or pharmacodynamics of tramadol include its transporters (adenosine triphosphate-binding cassette B1/multidrug resistance1/P-glycoprotein, organic cation transporter 1, serotonin transporter, and norepinephrine transporter) and receptor genes (mu1; see later discussion).[14] Given its mechanism of action, it is not surprising that 2 associated adverse reactions include seizures and serotonin syndrome. In regard to the metabolism of tramadol (through CYP2D6), some poor metabolizers have been found to have no response at all to tramadol. Poor metabolizers have also been shown to be mostly free of the adverse reactions of tramadol, whereas extensive metabolizers experience mild to moderate side effects. Ultrametabolizers, similar to codeine, can experience life-threatening side effects.[14]

STRONG OPIOIDS

Morphine

Morphine binds to the mu receptors resulting in an increase in the patients' pain threshold (see later discussion of mu-receptors). The active metabolite of morphine (morphine-6-glucuronide) is created by glucuronidation with the help of the hepatic isoenzyme UGT2B7. CYP2D6 only plays a minor role in morphine metabolism.[13] One of the adverse effects related to morphine is central respiratory depression. Morphine is subject to efflux by the P-glycoprotein transporter (encoded by ABCB1; also known as MDR1) along the blood-brain barrier.[15] Polymorphisms in ABCB1 can potentially affect blood-brain barrier transport of morphine and, therefore, show variability in the opioid effect on respiratory depression. One study showed that children with GG and GA genotypes of ABCB1 polymorphism (rs9282564) had a higher risk of respiratory depression, resulting in prolonged hospital stay.[15]

One study of 5 subjects with Gilbert syndrome (impaired glucuronidation secondary to a UGT1A1 polymorphism) did not show any differences in morphine clearance or plasma concentration when compared with controls.[16]

Another study examined 145 Italian subjects undergoing morphine therapy and found that pain relief variability was significantly associated with ABCB1 single-nucleotide polymorphism C3435T and the single-nucleotide polymorphism A80G of OPRM1. The association of these polymorphisms and pain relief in the study correlated into 3 groups (strong responders, responders, and nonresponders) with sensitivity close to 100% and specificity more than 70%.[17]

Diamorphine

Diamorphine (also known as heroin) is a common opioid-like drug that is known to be widely abused. Oral diamorphine has poor bioavailability secondary to its complete hepatic first-pass metabolism. It is catalyzed hepatically into 6-monoacetylmorphine and morphine.[18] One study shows that the CSNK1E single-nucleotide polymorphism (rs1534891) shows protection from diamorphine addiction. It has been implicated in negative regulation of sensitivity to opioids in rodents.[19]

Fentanyl

Fentanyl is a commonly used synthetic opioid that undergoes pulmonary first-pass metabolism, as well as hepatic metabolism, via CYP3A4.[20] One study in 2007 looked at 127 Korean subjects and the effect of fentanyl on respiratory rate under spinal anesthesia.[21] The study looked at 3 different single-nucleotide polymorphisms in ABCB1 (1236C> 2, 2677G > T/A, and 3435C > T) and found a trend suggesting ABCB1 polymorphisms may have clinical relevance in respiratory depression.

Given that CYP3A4 is involved in fentanyl metabolism, blood levels would be expected to rise in poor-metabolism patients receiving fentanyl.[22] One Japanese study evaluated the influence of both CYP3A4 and ABCB1 polymorphism on transdermal fentanyl pharmacokinetics and clinical responses in subjects who have cancer.[23] It obtained blood samples from 60 subjects 192 hours after starting transdermal fentanyl. Adverse effects, the need for rescue dosing, and clinical responses were evaluated. The measured fentanyl absorption rate was significantly higher in the CYP3A5*3/*3 group than in the *1/*1 and *1/*3 groups. This likely accounted for the greater incidence of central adverse events in the CYP3A5*3/*3 subjects than the *1/*1+*1/*3 subjects. ABCB1 1236 TT was found to be associated with decreased administration of rescue medication.

Buprenorphine

Buprenorphine is a semisynthetic opioid that is often coformulated with naloxone to prevent abuse in sublingual preparations.[13] Buprenorphine is metabolized by CYP3A4 in the liver to primarily norbuprenorphine.

OPRD1 (delta-opioid receptor; see later discussion) had previously been associated with heroin addiction and treatment outcomes. One study examined single-nucleotide polymorphisms (rs581111 and rs529520) to predict buprenorphine treatment outcomes for opioid dependence.[24] Female opioid addicts with GG genotype at rs581111 were found to have better outcomes when treated with buprenorphine compared with AG or AA genotype.

A recent study examined 107 subjects and the influence on gene polymorphisms on transdermal buprenorphine on pain control in subjects with critical limb ischemia.[25] Subjects who were AA homozygotes for CYP3A4 showed the best response to analgesic treatment.

Oxycodone and Oxymorphone

Oxycodone is a commonly prescribed analgesic with metabolites noroxycodone and oxymorphone (catalyzed by CYP3A4 and CYP2D6, respectively). Notably, noroxycodone has less than 1% of the analgesic properties of oxycodone.[6]

One study examined various effects of oxycodone on CYP2D6 polymorphisms.[26] Ultrametabolizers experienced a 1.5-fold to 6-fold increase in analgesic effects of oxycodone compared with extensive-metabolizers. Poor-metabolizers had 2-fold to 20-fold reduction of effects compared with extensive-metabolizers. The study went on to show that CYP3A inhibition showed a significant increase of oxycodone analgesic efficacy, as well as toxicity.

Given these large variations in clinical activity, urine or oral toxicology is now routinely performed on chronic pain patients for quantitative examination of metabolites.[6] This can give insight into the patients' specific enzyme activity. Patients with high levels of noroxycodone, for instance, and low oxymorphone levels are likely to be CYP2D6 deficient or have the enzyme inhibited.

OPIOID RECEPTORS

The 3 classic opioid receptors are known as mu, kappa, and delta and are coded for by the OPRM1, OPRK1, and OPRD1 genes, respectively. The largest genetic association study of opioid response examined a total of 112 single-nucleotide polymorphisms in 25 genes in more than 2200 subjects.[27] The genes examined included OPRM1, OPRK1, and OPRD1, and the investigation centered around their relationship to oral equivalent morphine doses. No association was identified with any of the single-nucleotide polymorphisms in this study. Nevertheless, there have been several association studies suggesting some relationship and further examining other opioids (see later discussion).

Mu-Opioid Receptor

The gene coding for the mu-opioid receptor is known as OPRM1. Gene knockout studies in mice have demonstrated that analgesic responses to opioids are primarily mediated by the mu-opioid receptor.[28]

Several single-nucleotide polymorphisms have been described in OPRM1. One of these OPRM1 single-nucleotide polymorphisms is A118G. One study found that subjects with chronic pain treated with opioids had a lower frequency of this polymorphism compared with opioid-naïve subjects.[29] This may suggest that this allele (G) is protective against pain. Another study explored epidural fentanyl and variations in OPRM1 alleles. Female subjects with G alleles (both heterozygous and homozygous) were found to have higher pressure pain thresholds than homozygous women with the more common A allele.[30]

However, this correlation of polymorphism to clinical opioid efficacy may not be so simple. One study examined the differences in morphine requirements over a 24-hour period for subjects with different alleles. The morphine was used for cancer pain relief and assessed 207 inpatients with stable morphine dosing over 3 days.[31] It suggests that OPRM1 GG genotypes required 93% higher morphine dose compared with AA genotypes. This may suggest that different opioids have varying effects on different alleles (**Table 2**).

Table 2
OPRM1 allele prevalence and morphine requirements for cancer pain relief

OPRM1 Genotype	Prevalence (%)	Average Morphine Requirement
AA	31.3	112 mg/24 h
AG	58.3	132 mg/24 h
GG	10.4	216 mg/24 h

Adapted from Liu YC, Wang WS. Human Mu-opioid Receptor Gene A118G Polymorphism Predicts the Efficacy of Tramadol/acetaminophen Combination Tablets (ultracet) in Oxaliplatin-induced Painful Neuropathy. Cancer 2012;118(6):1720; and Reyes-Gibby CC, Shete S, Rakvåg T, et al. Exploring Joint effects of genes and the clinical efficacy of morphine for cancer pain: OPRM1 and COMT Gene. Pain 2007;130(1–2):25–30.

Kappa-Opioid Receptor

The gene coding for the kappa-opioid receptor is known as OPRK1. The kappa-opioid receptor has been shown to produce aversive states, which are often used in preventing the development of opioid use reinforcement.[5] One examination of agonist-antagonist kappa opioids (ie, nalbuphine, pentazocine, and butorphanol) showed greater postoperative analgesia in female compared with male patients.[32]

Delta-Opioid Receptor

The gene coding for the delta-opioid receptor is known as OPRD1. One study examined OPRD1 polymorphisms and found them to be relevant for cocaine addiction in African American populations.[33] Another study reports an increased frequency of the minor G-allele of single-nucleotide polymorphism rs569356 in subjects with opioid dependence.[34]

CATECHOL-O-METHYLTRANSFERASE

Catechol-O-methyltransferase (COMT) metabolizes catecholamines and is associated with dopaminergic, adrenergic, noradrenergic, and serotonin neurotransmission.[5] It is estimated that up to 10% of variability in all pain sensitivity is associated with COMT single-nucleotide polymorphisms.

A study that examined the effect of COMT genes on predicting morphine requirements. Carriers of COMT Val/Val and Val/Met genotype were shown to require 63% and 23%, respectively, higher doses of morphine compared with carriers of the Met/Met genotype.[31]

One study examined 115 subjects of American Society of Anesthesiologists physical status I to III scheduled for radical gastrectomies under general anesthesia. The amount of fentanyl consumed and side effects were recorded for the first 24 to 48 hours postoperatively and each patient was screened for varying single-nucleotide polymorphisms of COMT.[35] Subjects with the haplotype ACCG consumed more fentanyl than GCGG and ATCA haplotypes during the first 24 and 48 hours after surgery. No differences were found between the incidence of nausea, vomiting, and dizziness among the single-nucleotide polymorphisms of the COMT gene.

One study examined the differences in mean pain score or dose intake of codeine in relation to various COMT polymorphisms. No significant differences were detected, although the study may not have been sufficiently powered to detect this between genotypic groups.[36]

KETAMINE

Ketamine is an antagonist for N-methyl-D-aspartate receptors and is widely used as an analgesic although it displays several other useful properties in anesthesia. There are several cytochrome enzymes that have been found to be involved in the N-demethylation of ketamine enantiomers. Some of these include CYP2B6, CYP2C9, and CYP3A4.[37] Review on the variability between CYP2D6 and CYP2C19 poor and extensive metabolizers found no differences in side effects of ketamine[38] although these cytochromes have not been previously identified to be involved in the metabolism of ketamine.[30] Further testing of 3A4 in a Swedish white population (comparing normal and slow metabolizers) showed no difference in the overall pharmacokinetics or in ketamine-related side effects.[38]

NONSTEROIDAL ANTI-INFLAMMATORY DRUGS

Nonsteroidal anti-inflammatory drugs (NSAIDs) are widely used nonopioid analgesics that act by inhibiting enzymes cyclooxygenase-1/2. These cyclooxygenase enzymes catalyze prostaglandin synthesis and, by this inhibition, NSAIDs ultimately provide anti-inflammatory, antipyretic and analgesic effects.[13] Some of the well-known harms of NSAIDs include its adverse effects on the cardiovascular and gastrointestinal system.

CYP2C9 polymorphisms may play a significant role toward these effects of NSAIDs.[39] NSAIDs used in analgesics (eg, flurbiprofen and celecoxib; **Table 3**) have been recommended to start treatment at half the normal recommended dose in poor metabolizers (CYP2C9*3/*3 genotype) to avoid adverse cardiovascular and gastrointestinal events.[39] These common variants (CYP2C9*2 and *3) of the CYP2C9 gene differ from the wild-type CYP2C9*1 allele by a single point mutation.[40] One case report describes a pediatric patient with an 8-fold higher area under the

Table 3
Nonsteroidal anti-inflammatory drugs metabolism and recommended dosing for pain

Type	Adverse Reaction	Polymorphism	Recommendation	Ethnicity
Celecoxib	Cardiovascular events	CYP2C9	Consider starting treatment at half the lowest recommended dose in poor metabolizers (CYP2C9*3/*3) to avoid adverse cardiovascular and gastrointestinal events	White
Flurbiprofen	Adverse cardiovascular, renal, and gastrointestinal events (including bleeding and ulceration)	CYP2C9	Poor metabolizers (CYP2C9*3/*3) should administrated with caution to avoid adverse cardiovascular and gastrointestinal events	White, Korean

Adapted from Ko TM, Wong CS, Wu JY, et al. Pharmacogenomics for Personalized Pain Medicine. Acta Anaesthesiol Taiwan 2016;54(1):26.

curve of celecoxib compared with an extensive metabolizer and was examined to be CYP2C9*3/*3.

CYP2C8 polymorphisms may also influence variability in pharmacokinetics of NSAIDS, more specifically ibuprofen and diclofenac. Polymorphisms in this enzyme have been shown to change the clearing capacity leading to abnormally higher levels.[41,42] CYP2C8 polymorphisms have also been implicated in gastrointestinal bleeds. One study examined the frequency of CYP2C8*3 allele in NSAID-induced gastrointestinal bleeds and found that it was significantly higher in NSAID users who experienced bleeds. This study also examined CYP2C9*2 and found that it also confers a higher risk of gastrointestinal bleed when taking NSAIDs.[43]

SUMMARY

Despite the potential for pharmacogenomics to improve patient care, there are still many barriers limiting its widespread use. Johnson[44] describes several commonly identified barriers to clinical implementation of pharmacogenomics in clinical practice. Some of these barriers include test turnaround time, cost of test or lack of reimbursement, and insufficient data. Despite these barriers, pharmacogenomics is slowly making its way into clinical practice.

One of the case reports previously described involving opioid poisoning in a breastfed infant prompted the FDA to change the codeine product label. It now includes information on the increased risk of morphine overdose in breastfed infants whose mothers are taking codeine and are ultrametabolizers.[45] Similarly, after the case report of the pediatric patient with an increased level of celecoxib secondary to being a poormetabolizer, the drug label for celecoxib now carries an FDA warning regarding CYP2C9 genotyping.[46]

It is clear that small but necessary steps are being made toward widespread clinical practice changes. Perhaps, someday, individualized care will be expanded through something as simple as noninvasive saliva testing.

REFERENCES

1. What Is Pharmacogenomics? Genetics Home Reference. Available at: https://ghr.nlm.nih.gov/primer/genomicresearch/pharmacogenomics. Accessed August 15, 2016.
2. Pain Research Funding Inadequate in the Face of Soaring Incidence and Treatment Costs. Press Room. Available at: http://americanpainsociety.org/about-us/press-room/pain-research-funding-inadequate. Accessed August 15, 2016.
3. US Food and Drug Administration. Preventable Adverse Drug Reactions: A Focus on Drug Interactions. Center for Drug Evaluation and Research. Available at: https://www.fda.gov/Drugs/DevelopmentApprovalProcess/DevelopmentResources/DrugInteractionsLabeling/ucm110632.htm. Accessed February 23, 2017.
4. Schug S, Ting S. The pharmacogenomics of pain management: prospects for personalized medicine. J Pain Res 2016;9:49–56.
5. Trescot AM, Faynboym S. A review of the role of genetic testing in pain medicine. Pain Physician 2014;17(5):425–45.
6. Trescot AM. Genetics and implications in perioperative analgesia. Best Pract Res Clin Anaesthesiol 2014;28(2):153–66.
7. Bradford LD. CYP2D6 Allele Frequency in European Caucasians, Asians, Africans and Their descendants. Pharmacogenomics 2002;3(2):229–43.
8. Linares OA, Fudin J, Schiesser WE, et al. CYP2D6 phenotype-specific codeine population pharmacokinetics. J Pain Palliat Care Pharmacother 2015;29(1):4–15.

9. Koren G, Cairns J, Chitayat D, et al. Pharmacogenetics of morphine poisoning in a breastfed neonate of a codeine-prescribed mother. Lancet 2006; 368(9536):704.
10. Gasche Y, Daali Y, Fathi M, et al. Codeine intoxication associated with ultrarapid CYP2D6 metabolism. N Engl J Med 2004;351(27):2827–31.
11. Barakat NH, Atayee RS, Best BM, et al. Relationship between the concentration of hydrocodone and its conversion to hydromorphone in chronic pain patients using urinary excretion data. J Anal Toxicol 2012 May;36(4):257–64.
12. Boswell MV, Stauble EM, Loyd GE, et al. The role of hydromorphone and OPRM1 in postoperative pain relief with hydrocodone. Pain Physician 2013;16(3):E227–35.
13. Kapur BM, Lala PK, Shaw JL. Pharmacogenetics of chronic pain management. Clin Biochem 2014;47(13–14):1169–87.
14. Lassen D, Damkier P, Brøsen K. The pharmacogenetics of tramadol. Clin Pharmacokinet 2015;54(8):825–36.
15. Sadhasivam S, Chidambaran V, Zhang X, et al. Opioid-induced respiratory depression: ABCB1 transporter pharmacogenetics. Pharmacogenomics J 2014;15(2): 119–26.
16. Skarke C, Schmidt H, Geisslinger G, et al. Pharmacokinetics of morphine are not altered in subjects with gilbert's syndrome. Br J Clin Pharmacol 2003;56(2): 228–31.
17. Campa D, Gioia A, Tomei A, et al. Association of ABCB1/MDR1 and OPRM1 gene polymorphisms with morphine pain relief. Clin Pharmacol Ther 2007;83(4): 559–66.
18. Kreek MJ. Pharmacogenetics and human molecular genetics of opiate and cocaine addictions and their treatments. Pharmacol Rev 2005;57(1):1–26.
19. Levran O, Peles E, Randesi M, et al. Dopaminergic pathway polymorphisms and heroin addiction: further support for association of CSNK1E variants. Pharmacogenomics 2014;15(16):2001–9.
20. Meyer MR, Maurer HH. Absorption, distribution, metabolism and excretion pharmacogenomics of drugs of abuse. Pharmacogenomics 2011;12(2):215–33.
21. Park H-J, Shinn HK, Ryu SH, et al. Genetic polymorphisms in the ABCB1 gene and the effects of fentanyl in koreans. Clin Pharmacol Ther 2006;81(4):539–46.
22. Kadiev E, Patel V, Rad P, et al. Role of pharmacogenetics in variable response to drugs: focus on opioids. Expert Opin Drug Metab Toxicol 2007;4(1):77–91.
23. Takashina Y, Naito T, Mino Y, et al. Impact of CYP3A5 and ABCB1 gene polymorphisms on fentanyl pharmacokinetics and clinical responses in cancer patients undergoing conversion to a transdermal system. Drug Metab Pharmacokinet 2012;27(4):414–21.
24. Clarke T-K, Crist RC, Ang A, et al. Genetic variation in OPRD1 and the response to treatment for opioid dependence with buprenorphine in European American females. Pharmacogenomics J 2013;14(3):303–8.
25. Blanco F, Muriel C, Labrador J, et al. Influence of UGT2B7, CYP3A4, and OPRM1 gene polymorphisms on transdermal buprenorphine pain control in patients with critical lower limb ischemia awaiting revascularization. Pain Pract 2016;16(7): 842–9.
26. Samer CF, Daali Y, Wagner M, et al. Genetic Polymorphisms and Drug Interactions Modulating CYP2D6 and CYP3A activities have a major effect on oxycodone analgesic efficacy and safety. Br J Pharmacol 2010;160(4):919–30.
27. Klepstad P, Fladvad T, Skorpen F, et al. Influence from genetic variability on opioid use for cancer pain: a European genetic association study of 2294 cancer pain patients. Pain 2011;152(5):1139–45.

28. Cregg R, Russo G, Gubbay A, et al. Pharmacogenetics of analgesic drugs. Br J Pain 2013;7(4):189–208.
29. Janicki PK, Schuler G, Francis D, et al. A genetic association study of the functional A118G polymorphism of the human mu-opioid receptor gene in patients with acute and chronic pain. Anesth Analg 2006;103(4):1011–7.
30. Fillingim RB, Kaplan L, Staud R, et al. The A118G single nucleotide polymorphism of the μ-opioid receptor gene (OPRM1) is associated with pressure pain sensitivity in humans. J Pain 2005;6(3):159–67.
31. Reyes-Gibby CC, Shete S, Rakvåg T, et al. Exploring joint effects of genes and the clinical efficacy of morphine for Cancer Pain: OPRM1 and COMT gene. Pain 2007;130(1):25–30.
32. Gear RW, Gordon NC, Hossaini-Zadeh M, et al. A subanalgesic dose of morphine eliminates nalbuphine anti-analgesia in postoperative pain. J Pain 2008;9(4):337–41.
33. Crist RC, Ambrose-Lanci LM, Vaswani M, et al. Case–control association analysis of polymorphisms in the delta-opioid receptor, OPRD1, with cocaine and opioid addicted populations. Drug Alcohol Depend 2013;127(1–3):122–8.
34. Zhang H, Gelernter J, Gruen JR, et al. Functional impact of a single-nucleotide polymorphism in the OPRD1 promoter region. J Hum Genet 2010;55(5):278–84.
35. Zhang F, Tong J, Hu J, et al. COMT gene haplotypes are closely associated with postoperative fentanyl dose in patients. Anesth Analg 2015;120(4):933–40.
36. Baber M, Chaudhry S, Kelly L, et al. The pharmacogenetics of codeine pain relief in the postpartum period. Pharmacogenomics J 2015;15(5):430–5.
37. Hijazi Y. Contribution of CYP3A4, CYP2B6, and CYP2C9 Isoforms to N-Demethylation of ketamine in human liver microsomes. Drug Metab Dispos 2002;30(7):853–8.
38. Persson J, Hasselström J, Maurset A, et al. Pharmacokinetics and Non-analgesic Effects of S- and R-ketamines in Healthy volunteers with normal and reduced metabolic capacity. Eur J Clin Pharmacol 2001;57(12):869–75.
39. Ko TM, Wong CS, Wu JY, et al. Pharmacogenomics for personalized pain medicine. Acta Anaesthesiol Taiwan 2016;54(1):24–30.
40. Yiannakopoulou E. Pharmacogenomics of acetylsalicylic acid and other nonsteroidal anti-inflammatory agents: clinical implications. Eur J Clin Pharmacol 2013;69(7):1369–73.
41. Martinez C, Garcia-Martin E, Blanco G, et al. The effect of the cytochrome P450 CYP2C8 polymorphism on the disposition of (R)-ibuprofen enantiomer in healthy subjects. Br J Clin Pharmacol 2005;59(1):62–8.
42. Kumar S. Extrapolation of diclofenac clearance from in vitro microsomal metabolism data: role of acyl glucuronidation and sequential oxidative metabolism of the acyl glucuronide. J Pharmacol Exp Ther 2002;303(3):969–78.
43. Blanco G, Martínez C, Ladero JM, et al. Interaction of CYP2C8 and CYP2C9 genotypes modifies the risk for nonsteroidal anti-inflammatory drugs-related acute gastrointestinal bleeding. Pharmacogenet Genomics 2008;18(1):37–43.
44. Johnson JA. Pharmacogenetics in Clinical Practice: How Far Have We Come and Where Are We Going? Pharmacogenomics 2013;14(7):835–43.
45. Crews KR, Gaedigk A, Dunnenberger HM, et al. Clinical pharmacogenetics implementation consortium (CPIC) Guidelines for codeine therapy in the context of cytochrome P450 2D6 (CYP2D6) genotype. Clin Pharmacol Ther 2011;91(2):321–6.
46. U.S. Food and Drug Administration. Table of Pharmacogenomic Biomarkers in Drug Labeling. Available at: https://www.fda.gov/Drugs/ScienceResearch/ResearchAreas/Pharmacogenetics/ucm083378.htm. Accessed February 23, 2017.

Novel Anticoagulant Agents in the Perioperative Setting

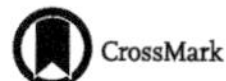

Allyson Lemay, MD[a], Alan D. Kaye, MD, PhD, DABA, DABPM, DABIPP[b], Richard D. Urman, MD, MBA[a,*]

KEYWORDS

- Anticoagulation • Novel oral anticoagulants • Regional anesthesia
- Neuraxial anesthesia • Perioperative management • ASRA guidelines

KEY POINTS

- An increasing number of oral anticoagulants have become available over the past decade. Each of these agents has differing implications on both regional and neuraxial anesthetic techniques.
- This article describes the pharmacology, pharmacokinetics, and pharmacodynamics of novel oral anticoagulants.
- It also describes the preoperative management of the novel oral anticoagulants and their implications for general and regional anesthesia.

INTRODUCTION

Novel oral anticoagulants (NOACs) have increased in popularity and use over the past 10 years (**Table 1**). They are approved for use for prevention of stroke in nonvalvular atrial fibrillation, deep vein thrombosis (DVT)/pulmonary embolism (PE) treatment, and prophylaxis for DVT for some surgical procedures. NOACs were introduced as a replacement for warfarin because they are the first oral anticoagulants that do not require frequent laboratory monitoring. On the downside, compared with warfarin, there are no specific reversal agents for bleeding and there is also a lack of randomized controlled trials showing safety in the timing of surgical procedures and regional anesthetic techniques. At present, guidelines are based mostly on drug half-life and other limited data. As a result, there continue to be differing opinions about discontinuation of NOACs in the published literature. In this comprehensive review we describe

Disclosure: The authors have nothing to disclose.
[a] Department of Anesthesiology, Perioperative and Pain Medicine, Harvard Medical School, Brigham and Women's Hospital, 75 Francis Street, Boston, MA 02115, USA; [b] Department of Anesthesiology and Pain Medicine, Louisiana State University School of Medicine, LSU Health Science Center, 1542 Tulane Avenue, Room 659, New Orleans, LA 70112, USA
* Corresponding author.
E-mail address: urmanr@gmail.com

Anesthesiology Clin 35 (2017) 305–313
http://dx.doi.org/10.1016/j.anclin.2017.01.016
1932-2275/17/
anesthesiology.theclinics.com

Table 1
Novel oral anticoagulants

Direct Thrombin Inhibitor	Factor Xa Inhibitors	Antiplatelet Agents (P2Y12 Receptor Antagonists)
• Dabigatran	• Rivaroxaban • Apixaban • Edoxaban • Betrixaban	• Clopidogrel • Prasugrel • Ticagrelor

the pharmacology and pharmacokinetics of the NOACs and discuss implications for perioperative care.

DIRECT THROMBIN INHIBITORS

Dabigatran Etexilate

Dabigatran etexilate is currently the only oral direct thrombin inhibitor on the market. It has been approved for prevention of stroke in nonvalvular atrial fibrillation, treatment of acute venous thromboembolism (VTE), and prevention of VTE after total joint surgery. Dabigatran etexilate is an oral prodrug that is rapidly absorbed in the stomach, with peak plasma concentrations reached within 2 hours,[1] and then converted to its active form, dabigatran. Its bioavailability is estimated at about 7%.[2] It reversibly binds to thrombin to inhibit its activity in the coagulation cascade and prevent the formation of fibrin from fibrinogen and also prevents activation of factors V, VIII, and X. Following absorption, dabigatran undergoes rapid redistribution and has an elimination half-life of 12 to 17 hours in healthy adults.[1] In patients with end-stage renal disease, the half-life is prolonged to approximately 28 hours.[3] Therefore, the dose should be adjusted for renal function and if creatinine clearance is estimated to be less than 30 mL/min, dabigatran use is contraindicated.[4] It does not undergo metabolism by the cytochrome P (CYP) 450 system and undergoes 80% renal excretion and 20% gastrointestinal (GI) excretion.[5] Moderate hepatic impairment has not been shown to affect the pharmacokinetics of dabigatran and therefore these patients do not require a dose adjustment.[6]

At present the only reversal techniques available for dabigatran include hemodialysis and activated charcoal administered within 1 to 2 hours of oral dosing. Idarucizumab, an antibody fragment that is specific in the reversal of dabigatran, is currently undergoing testing and clinical trials. Small studies have shown complete reversal of dabigatran within minutes of administration of idarucizumab and it is currently undergoing clinical trials.[7]

FACTOR XA INHIBITORS

There are currently 4 available orally active factor Xa inhibitors on the market with more in development. Direct factor Xa inhibitors work by binding to free factor Xa and factor Xa bound to the prothrombinase complex and therefore interrupt both the intrinsic and extrinsic coagulation cascade, preventing the ultimate formation of thrombin.

Rivaroxaban

Rivaroxaban was the first available orally active factor Xa inhibitor. In the United States, it is currently approved for use in prevention of VTE and stroke in patients with nonvalvular atrial fibrillation, treatment of VTE, and for the prevention of VTE after orthopedic surgery. It has also been shown to have benefit in patients with recent acute coronary syndromes. When rivaroxaban was added to a standard antiplatelet therapy, there was a significant reduction in the composite end point of death from myocardial infarction (MI), stroke, and other cardiovascular causes.[8]

Rivaroxaban has a rapid onset with peak plasma concentrations within 2.5 to 4 hours of oral dosing. In healthy patients, maximum inhibition of factor Xa occurs at approximately 3 hours with effects lasting up to 12 hours.[9] Once absorbed, greater than 90% of the drug is protein bound and it has a small volume of distribution. The terminal half-life of rivaroxaban was shown to be 5.7 to 9.2 hours, but this can be prolonged in elderly patients because of age-related declines in renal function.[9,10] Hepatic metabolism does occur and involves CYP3A4-independent, CYP2C8-independent, and CYP-independent mechanisms to form inactive metabolites.[11] Therefore, rivaroxaban is contraindicated in patients with severe liver disease. Elimination occurs by renal excretion and biliary/fecal excretion of unmetabolized drug. In patients with creatinine clearance less than 30 mL/min, rivaroxaban is contraindicated. In healthy patients, it has been shown that the pharmacokinetics of rivaroxaban are not significantly affected by sex or age.[12]

Monitoring of rivaroxaban is not standardized but is best achieved by monitoring anti-factor Xa levels or prothrombin time (PT). It prolongs the PT but prolongation only occurs during peak drug concentrations and there may be only minimal prolongations during steady state.[13] International Normalized Ratio (INR), activated partial thromboplastin time (aPTT), and ecarin clotting time are not reliable ways to measure the anticoagulant effect of rivaroxaban.

Reversal of rivaroxaban can be achieved by active charcoal if given within 8 hours of ingestion or with 4-factor prothrombin complex, which has been shown to reverse the anticoagulant effects of the drug in healthy individuals.[14] There has also been recent studies on Andexanat which shows promise as a rapidly acting reversal of direct Factor Xa inhibitors. It is currently in clinical trial to evaluate both efficacy and safety.[15]

Apixaban

Apixaban is another oral factor Xa inhibitor that is currently on the market. Apixaban is approved in the United States for use to decrease stroke risk in patients with nonvalvular atrial fibrillation as well as for prophylaxis and treatment of patients with PE. In the 2013 Apixaban for the Initial Management of Pulmonary Embolism and Deep-Vein Thrombosis as First-Line Therapy (AMPLIFY) trial, apixaban was shown to be noninferior in preventing recurrent VTE and showed a decrease in all-cause hospitalizations.[16]

Apixaban has a rapid onset with peak concentrations at approximately 3 to 4 hours of oral dosing. It has approximately a 50% bioavailability in the GI tract and most of the drug is protein bound and therefore nondialyzable. The half-life of apixaban is approximately 12 hours and, like other NOACs, the half-life is prolonged in patients with renal disease. Apixaban is metabolized hepatically, mainly through the CYP3A4 system, and is eliminated mainly through the biliary system (75%) with some renal excretion (25%).

Apixaban prolongs the PT/INR and aPTT and this relationship has been shown to be dosage dependent, with increasing oral doses causing a greater effect on laboratory values.[17] Given the high variability of laboratory values to consistent oral dosing, the values do not accurately reflect the pharmacodynamics of the drug and therefore are not used routinely for monitoring. Factor Xa assays have shown high sensitivity regarding the anticoagulation effect of apixaban but it is still not routinely used for monitoring.

Edoxaban

Edoxaban, one of the newest of the direct Xa inhibitor family, has been studied for use in reducing stroke risk in nonvalvular atrial fibrillation. The Effective Anticoagulation

With Factor Xa Next Generation in Atrial Fibrillation–Thrombolysis in Myocardial Infarction (ENGAGE-AF TIMI) trial compared the use of edoxaban with that of warfarin for stroke prevention in nonvalvular atrial fibrillation and found it to be noninferior in the prevention of stroke and systemic embolism, with a significantly lower bleeding risk and decreased death rate from cardiovascular causes.[18] The Hokusai VTE trial compared edoxaban use with warfarin for VTE prevention and showed edoxaban to be noninferior to warfarin with a significantly lower bleeding risk.[19]

Edoxaban is rapidly absorbed and reaches a maximum plasma level at approximately 1 to 2 hours after oral absorption and steady state is reached at about 3 days.[20] It binds approximately 50% of plasma proteins, with the rest remaining unbound in the plasma.[21] It has an approximate half life of 10–14 hours. Metabolism of the drug is mainly through hydrolysis but the CYP3A4 system also has a minor contribution.[22] Excretion mainly involves the GI tract (approximately 62%) and renal system (approximately 35%).[22] A decrease in renal function has been shown to prolong the half-life of edoxaban, and dose adjustments may be considered in these patient populations.[23] Edoxaban is not cleared by hemodialysis and therefore dialysis-dependent patients do not require dose adjustments.[24] A mild or moderate decline in hepatic function does not significantly affect the half-life of edoxaban, and dose adjustments are not required.[25]

Edoxaban has been shown to prolong the PT after administration but both the INR and partial thromboplastin time have not been shown to be sensitive tests for monitoring the anticoagulation activity of edoxaban.[26] Anti-Xa level is considered the best test for monitoring anticoagulation quantification, but is not required or routinely used.[26] Although there are no specific guidelines from the American Society of Regional Anesthesia and Pain Medicine (ASRA), some institutional guidelines recommend holding edoxaban until at least 3 days prior to spinal or epidural placement.

Betrixaban

Betrixaban is a direct factor Xa inhibitor that is currently in phase III clinical trials comparing its effectiveness with other anticoagulants in orthopedic thromboprophylaxis as well as stroke prevention in nonvalvular atrial fibrillation.

Betrixaban has rapid oral absorption with peak concentrations at about 3 to 4 hours after administration.[27] Food that is high in fat seems to affect oral absorption and has been shown to decrease the peak concentration by up to 50%.[28] Approximately 60% of betrixaban is bound to plasma proteins and the half-life of the drug is about 20 hours.[28] Excretion is mainly through the hepatobiliary system (approximately 82%–89%) and it has been shown to have the smallest percentage of renal clearance among all of the direct factor Xa oral anticoagulants.[27] Given the lack of renal excretion, betrixaban could prove to be the safest NOAC to use in patients with impaired renal function.

Like the other NOACs, both INR and PTT are insensitive tests to determine the anticoagulant effect of betrixaban, while the anti-Xa assay is likely the best test to determine the anticoagulation status of the patient.[28]

NOVEL ORAL ANTICOAGULANTS AND REGIONAL ANESTHESIA

Anticoagulants are the main risk factor for hemorrhagic complications following neuraxial anesthesia.[29] Therefore, patients on anticoagulants provide an increased concern for anesthesiologists when determining whether or not a regional anesthetic technique is appropriate. Older anticoagulants such warfarin and enoxaparin have been well studied and have sensitive laboratory tests to determine the anticoagulation status of the patient, making the decision to perform regional anesthesia is more straightforward. ASRA sets forth specific guidelines for anticoagulants using both laboratory values and timing of last anticoagulant dose as the basis for appropriateness of regional anesthetic use (**Table 2**).[30] However, the newer oral anticoagulants, as discussed earlier, do not have sensitive laboratory tests to determine the patient's anticoagulation status and therefore it makes it more difficult to set forth guidelines on how long these anticoagulants should be stopped before neuraxial anesthesia is considered.

For the NOACs, it has been proposed that using the drug's elimination half-life is the most effective way to determine the safety of the timing of regional anesthesia. Most guidelines use approximately 2-3 elimination half-lives as the time needed between discontinuation of the drug and the regional technique.[31]

The 2015 ASRA guidelines have specific recommendations for some of the oral anticoagulants that were discussed earlier. They recommend that rivaroxaban be discontinued for 3 days before interventional pain procedures, neuraxial puncture, or catheter manipulation, and withholding the medication until 24 hours after the procedure is performed. It is recommended that apixaban be withheld for 3 to 5 days and for 24 hours after the procedure is performed. It is recommended that dabigatran be withheld for 4 to 5 days unless the patient has impaired renal function, in which case it should be held for 6 days and for 24 hours after the procedure is performed. There are no specific ASRA guidelines for edoxaban or betrixaban. The ASRA guidelines use approximately 5 half-lives when determining drug discontinuation, which is much longer than the 2-3 half-lives proposed by other professional societies.

Given the lack of research on safety of regional anesthesia with NOACs, anesthesiologists must consider whether the benefit outweighs the risk when determining whether a regional technique is appropriate for each patient.

ANTIPLATELET AGENTS

Oral antiplatelet agents have multiple clinical indications, including patients with coronary artery disease with previous stenting, peripheral vascular disease, or prior cerebral vascular accidents. Most commonly they are used in conjunction with aspirin to impair platelet function and prevent thrombosis. Clopidogrel, ticagrelor, and prasugrel are antiplatelet agents that work by inhibiting the ADP receptors on platelet surfaces. Specifically, these agents are P2Y12 receptor antagonists, which irreversibly bind the

Table 2
American Society of Regional Anesthesia (ASRA) recommendations for time to hold novel oral anticoagulants before neuraxial anesthesia

Drug	Days to Hold Before Neuraxial Anesthesia
Dabigatran	5
Rivaroxaban	3
Apixaban	3
Edoxaban	No recommendation
Betrixaban	No recommendation
Clopidogrel	7
Prasugrel	7–10

Data from Horlocker TT, Wedel DJ, Rowlingson JC, et al. Regional anesthesia in the patient receiving antithrombotic or thrombolytic therapy: American Society of Regional Anesthesia and Pain Medicine Evidence-Based Guidelines (Third Edition). Reg Anesth Pain Med 2010;35(1):64–101.

receptor to prevent ADP binding. This action reduces platelet function and prevents platelet aggregation. These agents have significant anesthetic implications for both general and regional techniques.

Clopidogrel

Clopidogrel is one of the most commonly used antiplatelet agents on the market, second only to aspirin. It is a second-generation thienopyridine and in the Clopidogrel versus Aspirin in Patients at Risk of Ischaemic Events (CAPRIE) trial clopidogrel was shown to be more effective than aspirin in reducing the risks of MI, ischemic stroke, and vascular mortality, while having a similar safety profile.[32] Clopidogrel is a prodrug that must be activated in vivo by a 2-step process requiring CYP450, CYP3A, and CYP2C19 enzymes.[33] Genetic polymorphism and differences in oral absorption make both the pharmacokinetics and pharmacodynamics of clopidogrel extremely variable. Because of genetic differences in the CYP system, up to about 15% of patients have an inadequate platelet inhibitory response to clopidogrel and are at high risk for in-stent thrombosis. Clopidogrel is highly protein bound and has approximately even excretion through the GI tract and renal system.[34]

Prasugrel

Prasugrel is an irreversible P2Y12 receptor antagonist and part of the thienopyridine family, which has been shown to decrease cardiovascular-related death in nonfatal MI compared with dual antiplatelet therapy, without demonstrating a higher risk of major bleeding.[35] It is a prodrug that requires enzymatic metabolism through the CYP450 system to achieve its antiplatelet action but, unlike clopidogrel, it only requires a 1-step metabolic activation. It is initially hydrolyzed in the GI tract to thiolactone and then converted to its active metabolite.[36] Prasugrel has peak plasma concentrations approximately 30 minutes after absorption and has a long duration of action (about 3 days).[37] Approximately 98% of the drug is bound to albumin and it is excreted mainly through the kidneys and GI tract.[36]

Ticagrelor

Ticagrelor is an orally active reversible P2Y12 receptor antagonist and part of the cyclopentyl triazolopyrimidine family. In the 2009 Platelet Inhibition and Patient Outcomes (PLATO) trial it was shown to have lower rate of death form vascular causes, MI, or stroke without a significant difference in overall major bleeding.[38] It is orally absorbed and does not require enzymatic activation, which therefore removes the patient pharmacokinetics variability as a issue, which is seen with clopidogrel. It also has a more rapid onset of platelet inhibition compared with clopidogrel and has been shown to have peak platelet inhibition at approximately 2 to 4 hours[39] with a terminal half-life of 7 hours.[40]

ANTIPLATELET AGENTS AND REGIONAL ANESTHESIA

Given the increased bleeding risk of patients on antiplatelet agents, certain guidelines are in place to aid in determining the safety of regional and neuraxial anesthetic techniques. ASRA has specific recommendations based on the pharmacokinetics of each of the antiplatelet agents. Specifically, it recommends stopping Plavix 7 days before, stopping prasugrel 7 to 10 days before, and stopping ticagrelor 5 to 7 days before performing neuraxial or regional anesthesia[30] (see **Table 2**). An individualized cost-benefit analysis should be performed based on the patient's risk of bleeding and in-stent thrombosis versus the benefit of a regional technique. In patients with unstable angina on dual antiplatelet therapy with aspirin and clopidogrel, ASRA recommends only stopping the clopidogrel 5 days before, as long as the patient presents a higher risk of perioperative cardiac events.[30] Specific platelet function assays can be done to determine return of normal platelet function, but they are not routinely performed. Anesthesiologists must use the ASRA guidelines, cardiologist's recommendations, and their own clinical judgment in determining the safety of regional or neuraxial anesthesia in anticoagulated patients.

SUMMARY

As oral anticoagulants grow in popularity, understanding of the pharmacology and pharmacokinetics becomes increasingly important to anesthesiologists in the perioperative setting. Current guidelines on the NOACs as well as personal clinical judgment should be used to determine the safety of regional and neuraxial anesthetic techniques. With future research and increasing outcomes data available to the practitioners, the current guidelines may change over time to better reflect the anticoagulation status of patients and safe practices.

REFERENCES

1. Stangier J, Rathgen K, Stähle H, et al. The pharmacokinetics, pharmacodynamics and tolerability of dabigatran etexilate, a new oral direct thrombin inhibitor, in healthy male subjects. Br J Clin Pharmacol 2007;64(3):292–302.
2. Blech S, Ebner T, Ludwig-Schwellinger E, et al. The metabolism and disposition of the oral direct thrombin inhibitor, dabigatran, in humans. Drug Metab Dispos 2008;36(2):386–99.
3. Stangier J, Rathgen K, Stähle H, et al. Influence of renal impairment on the pharmacokinetics and pharmacodynamics of oral dabigatran etexilate: an open-label, parallel-group, single-centre study. Clin Pharmoacokinet 2010;49(4):259–68.
4. Wittkowsky A. New oral anticoagulants: a practical guide for clinicians. J Thromb Thrombolysis 2010;29(2):182–91.
5. Stangier J, Clemens A. Pharmacology, pharmacokinetics, and pharmacodynamics of dabigatran etexilate, an oral direct thrombin inhibitor. Clin Appl Thromb Hemost 2009;15(Suppl 1):9S–16S.
6. Stangier J, Stahle H, Rathgen K, et al. Pharmacokinetics and pharmacodynamics of dabigatran etexilate, an oral direct thrombin inhibitor, are not affected by moderate hepatic impairment. J Clin Pharmacol 2008;48(12):1411–9.
7. Pollack CV, Reilly PA, Eikelboom J, et al. Idarucizumab for dabigatran reversal. N Engl J Med 2015;373(6):511–20.
8. Mega JL, Braunwald E, Wiviott SD, et al. Rivaroxaban in patients with a recent acute coronary syndrome. N Engl J Med 2012;366(1):9–19.
9. Kubitza D, Becka M, Wensing G, et al. Safety, pharmacodynamics, and pharmacokinetics of BAY 59-7939—an oral, direct factor Xa inhibitor—after multiple dosing in healthy male subjects. Eur J Clin Pharmacol 2005;61(12):873–80.
10. Kubitza D, Becka M. Dose-escalation study of the pharmacokinetics and pharmacodynamics of rivaroxaban in healthy elderly subjects. Curr Med Res Opin 2008;24(10):2757–65.
11. Gross PL, Weitz JI. New anticoagulants for treatment of venous thromboembolism. Arterioscler Thromb Vasc Biol 2008;28(3):380–6.
12. Kubitza D, Becka M, Roth A, et al. The influence of age and gender on the pharmacokinetics and pharmacodynamics of rivaroxaban—an oral, direct factor Xa inhibitor. J Clin Pharmacol 2013;53(3):249–55.

13. Eriksson BL, Quinlan DJ, Weitz JI, et al. Comparative pharmacodynamics and pharmacokinetics of oral direct thrombin and factor Xa inhibitors in development. Clin Pharmacokinet 2009;48(1):1–22.
14. Mivares MA, Davis K. Newer oral anticoagulants: a review of laboratory monitoring options and reversal agents in the hemorrhagic patient. Am J Health Syst Pharm 2012;69(17):1473–84.
15. Siegal DM, Curnutte JT, Connolly SJ, et al. Andexanet alpha for the reversal of factor Xa inhibitor activity. N Engl J Med 2015;373:2413–24.
16. Liu X, Johnson M, Mardekian J, et al. Apixaban reduces hospitalizations in patients with venous thromboembolism: an analysis of the Apixaban for the Initial Management of Pulmonary Embolism and Deep-Vein Thrombosis at First-Line Therapy (AMPLIFY) trial. J Am Heart Assoc 2015;4(12) [pii:e002340].
17. Frost C, Wang J, Nepal S, et al. Apixaban, an oral, direct factor Xa inhibitor: single dose safety, pharmacokinetics, pharmacodynamics and food effect in healthy subjects. Br J Clin Pharmacol 2013;75(2):476–87.
18. Giugliano RP, Ruff CT, Braunwald E, et al. Edoxaban versus warfarin in patients with atrial fibrillations. N Engl J Med 2013;369(22):2093–104.
19. Hokusai-VTE Investigators, Buller HR, Décousus H, Grosso MA, et al. Edoxaban versus warfarin for the treatment of symptomatic venous thromboembolism. N Engl J Med 2013;369(15):1406–15.
20. Matsushima N, Lee F, Sato T, et al. Bioavailability and safety of the factor Xa inhibitor edoxaban and the effects of quinidine in healthy subjects. Clin Pharmacol Drug Dev 2013;2(4):358–66.
21. Ogata K, Mendell-Harary J, Tachibana M, et al. Clinical safety, tolerability, pharmacokinetics, and pharmacodynamics of the novel factor Xa inhibitor edoxaban in healthy volunteers. J Clin Pharmacol 2010;50(7):743–53.
22. Bathala MS, Masumoto H, Oguma T, et al. Pharmacokinetics, biotransformation, and mass balance of edoxaban, a selective, direct factor Xa inhibitor, in humans. Drug Metab Dispos 2012;40(12):2250–5.
23. Switzer MP, Wani P, Gosavi S, et al. Clinical pharmacology and role of edoxaban in contemporary antithrombotic therapy. Cardiovasc Hematol Agents Med Chem 2015;13(2):98–104.
24. Parasrampuria DA, Marbury T, Matsushima N, et al. Pharmacokinetics, safety, and tolerability of edoxaban in end-stage renal disease subjects undergoing haemodialysis. Thromb Haemost 2015;113(4):719–27.
25. Mendell J, Johnson L, Chen S, et al. An open-label, phase 1 study to evaluate the effects of hepatic impairment on edoxaban pharmacokinetics and pharmacodynamics. J Clin Pharmacol 2015;55(12):1395–405.
26. Cuker A, Husseinzadeh H. Laboratory measurement of the anticoagulant activity of edoxaban: a systematic review. J Thromb Thrombolysis 2015;39(3):288–94.
27. Turpie AG, Bauer KA, Davidson BL, et al. A randomized evaluation of betrixaban, an oral factor Xa inhibitor, for prevention of thromboembolic events after total knee replacement (EXPERT). Thromb Haemost 2009;101(1):68–76.
28. Chan NC, Bhagirath V, Eikelboom JW, et al. Profile of betrixaban and its potential in the prevention and treatment of venous thromboembolism. Vasc Health Risk Manag 2015;11:343–51.
29. Lee LA, Posner KL, Domino KB, et al. Injuries associated with regional anesthesia in the 1980s and 1990s: a closed claim analysis. Anesthesiology 2004;101(1): 143–52.
30. Horlocker TT, Wedel DJ, Rowlingson JC, et al. Regional anesthesia in the patient receiving antithrombotic or thrombolytic therapy: American Society of Regional

Anesthesia and pain medicine evidence-based guidelines (third edition). Reg Anesth Pain Med 2010;35(1):64–101.
31. Gogarten W, Vandermeulen E, Van Aken H, et al. Regional anaesthesia and antithrombotic agents: recommendations of the European Society of Anaesthesiology. Eur J Anaesthesiol 2010;27(12):999–1015.
32. CAPRIE Steering Committee. A randomised, blinded, trial of clopidogrel versus aspirin in patients at risk of ischaemic events (CAPRIE). Lancet 1996; 348(9038):1329–39.
33. Collet JP, Hulot JS, Pena A, et al. Cytochrome P450 2C19 polymorphism in young patients treated with clopidogrel after myocardial infarction: a cohort study. Lancet 2009;373(9660):309–17.
34. Lins R, Broekhuysen J, Necciari J, et al. Pharmacokinetic profile of 14C-labeled clopidogrel. Semin Thromb Hemost 1999;25(Suppl 2):29–33.
35. Wiviott SD, Braunweld E, McCabe CH, et al. Prasugrel versus clopidogrel in patients with acute coronary syndromes. N Engl J Med 2007;357(20):2001–15.
36. Farid NA, Smith RL, Gillespie TA, et al. The disposition of prasugrel, a novel thienopyridine, in humans. Drug Metab Dispos 2007;35(7):1096–104.
37. Sugidachi A, Asai F, Ogawa T, et al. The in vivo pharmacological profile of CS-747, a novel antiplatelet agent with platelet ADP receptor antagonist properties. Br J Pharmacol 2000;129(7):1439–46.
38. Wallentin L, Becker RC, Budaj A, et al. Ticagrelor versus clopidogrel in patients with acute coronary syndromes. N Engl J Med 2009;361(11):1045–57.
39. Husted S, Emanuelsson H, Heptinstall S, et al. Pharmacodynamics, pharmacokinetics, and safety of the oral reversible P2Y12 antagonist AZD6140 with aspirin in patients with atherosclerosis: a double-blind comparison to clopidogrel with aspirin. Eur Heart J 2006;27(9):1038–47.
40. Teng R, Butler K. Pharmacokinetics, pharmacodynamics, tolerability and safety of the single ascending doses of ticagrelor, a reversibly binding oral P2Y(12) receptor antagonist, in healthy subjects. Eur J Clin Pharmacol 2010;66(5):487–96.

Pharmacologic Properties of Novel Local Anesthetic Agents in Anesthesia Practice

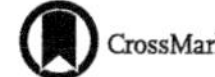

Chih H. King, MD, PhD[a], Sascha S. Beutler, MD, PhD[a],
Alan D. Kaye, MD, PhD, DABA, DABPM, DABIPP[b], Richard D. Urman, MD, MBA[a,*]

KEYWORDS

- Local anesthetics • Delivery systems • Site-1 sodium channel blockers • Adjuvants
- Liposomal bupivacaine • Proliposomal ropivacaine • Tetrodotoxin • Neosaxitoxin
- Bupivacaine

KEY POINTS

- Duration of traditional amide-based and ester-based local anesthetics when used in peripheral blocks is limited to a few hours.
- Several new approaches to extending the therapeutic duration of peripheral blocks are available or are currently under development.
- Naturally occurring site-1 selective sodium channel blockers can provide longer peripheral blocks, while limiting neurologic or cardiac toxicity.
- Various local anesthetics delivery systems can provide longer block duration, lower postoperative pain, lower opioid requirement, lower hospital cost, and/or repeatable triggered local anesthetics release.
- Novel adjuvants of local anesthetics, such as magnesium and dexmedetomidine, can extend peripheral block duration and lower postoperative opioid requirement.

INTRODUCTION

Local anesthetics (LAs) are part of the multimodal approach to provide intraoperative and postoperative pain management. However, the duration of traditional amide-based and ester-based LAs is normally limited to only a few hours. Techniques, such as continuous catheter placement or multiple serial injections, can be used to enhance the duration and effect of LAs for postoperative pain control. However, these

Disclosure of Relationship with Commercial Company: The authors have nothing to disclose.

[a] Department of Anesthesiology, Perioperative and Pain Medicine, Brigham and Women's Hospital, 75 Francis Street, Boston, MA 02115, USA; [b] Department of Anesthesiology and Pain Medicine, Louisiana State University School of Medicine, LSU Health Science Center, 1542 Tulane Avenue, Room 659, New Orleans, LA 70112, USA
* Corresponding author.
E-mail address: rurman@partners.org

Anesthesiology Clin 35 (2017) 315–325
http://dx.doi.org/10.1016/j.anclin.2017.01.019

approaches increase the risk of infection, toxicity, and cost. Therefore, alternative methods of extending the clinical duration of nerve blocks have always been a topic of significant interest. This article focuses on 3 newer approaches to extending the therapeutic duration of peripheral blocks:

1. Site-1 sodium channel blockers, such as tetrodotoxin (TTX) and neosaxitoxin (NeoSTX)
2. Novel LA delivery systems
3. The adjuvants, magnesium and dexmedetomidine.

NATURALLY OCCURRING SITE-1 SELECTIVE SODIUM CHANNEL BLOCKERS

NeoSTX and TTX are selective sodium channel blockers that are naturally produced by animals such as pufferfish and shellfish. Both substances have been used for decades in laboratory as a pharmacologic tool to selectively block and study a subset of sodium channels, specifically the voltage-gated sodium channels Nav1.1, Nav1.3, Nav1.6, and Nav1.7.[1] These compounds have a different mechanism of action than lidocaine. Specifically, they interact with the extracellular aspect of the α-subunit of the voltage-gated sodium channel and thus can act in a synergistic manner with traditional LAs.[2–4] Notably, there are subtypes of the TTX-sensitive voltage-gated sodium channels that are preferentially expressed in peripheral neurons (eg, Nav1.7 in dorsal root ganglion and sympathetic neurons). This may open up the possibility of blocking peripheral pain conduction without affecting cardiac or central nervous system electrical conduction.[1] For example, patients with specific mutations in Nav1.7 show a severely impaired pain perception from birth but are otherwise normal, including having a normal proprioception, temperature sensation, and sympathetic response.[5] Selective naturally occurring sodium channel blockers, such as NeoSTX and TTX, have come into renewed attention because traditional amide-based and ester-based LAs do not reliably provide analgesia beyond 6 to 12 hours via single-shot injection.[6] Also, intravascular injection or excessive dosage of traditional LAs can cause neurologic or cardiac toxicity. In contrast, toxicities from NeoSTX and TTX are primarily due to diaphragmatic paralysis and respiratory failure, which are reversible.

Among the selective sodium channel blockers, NeoSTX has been demonstrated to be the most potent both in vitro and in vivo.[7,8] It differs from saxitoxin (STX) by the addition of 1 oxygen atom.[9] Like the other substances in this family, NeoSTX is a site-1 sodium channel blocker that selectively binds to the outer pore of the voltage-gated sodium channels, interrupting the depolarization of excitable cells and propagation of action potential.[10] Unlike traditional LAs, in studies of anesthetized animals NeoSTX seemed to be devoid of cardiotoxicity.[11] An overdose of NeoSTX produces reversible skeletal and respiratory muscle weakness, which can be treated with respiratory support until the patient makes full recovery. This lack of significant cardiac effect may be secondary to the extremely low binding affinity of cardiac Purkinje fibers to selective sodium blockers.[12] In addition, although TTX can cause substantial hypotension via direct action on smooth muscle cells and sympathetic nerves, this is less of an issue with STX-related compound.[13] Similar to LAs, the addition of vasoconstrictors, such as epinephrine, can help reduce systemic concentration levels, which results in improved potency and duration while decreasing systemic toxicity.[14]

More recently, multiple in vivo studies and randomized clinical trials have examined the LAs properties and safety profile of NeoSTX. In randomized studies of healthy male subjects, subcutaneous injection of NeoSTX produced a significantly longer effect on pain threshold compared with bupivacaine, which was increased even further by the coinjection of epinephrine. Notably, none of the volunteers reported any motor disability or discomfort that was associated with NeoSTX or with the combination of NeoSTX and epinephrine.[14] In another randomized double-blinded study of subjects following laparoscopic cholecystectomy, the NeoSTX group had lower median pain score at rest and with movement 12 hours postoperatively compared with the bupivacaine group. There was no difference in adverse event rate between the bupivacaine and NeoSTX group.[15] Finally, in a phase 1 double-blind block-randomized controlled trial, the combination of NeoSTX with bupivacaine and epinephrine was also found to exhibit longer block duration (almost 5-fold longer) compared with bupivacaine, NeoSTX alone, or saline. Healthy male subjects who received subcutaneous infiltration of NeoSTX with bupivacaine did not experience increased serious adverse events versus bupivacaine alone, although perioral numbness and tingling were noted at higher doses, which were significantly reduced by the addition of epinephrine.[16]

Another potent sodium channel blocker, TTX, which has quite similar pharmacokinetics to STX, has also received attention for having potential application as an LA with minimal myotoxicity[17,18] and neurotoxicity,[19] while showing marked synergism with conventional ester and amide LAs in producing prolonged block duration in multiple animal studies. For example, when used alone in a rat sciatic nerve block, TTX or bupivacaine each produces approximately 150 minutes of block duration but when injected together they produce a block duration of 570 minutes.[20] Similar to NeoSTX, coinjection of epinephrine reduced the median effective concentration of TTX for nociception while prolonging its duration, thereby quadrupling the therapeutic index of TTX.[7] Finally, a study examined the effect of TTX on persistent muscle pain by analyzing the effect of TTX injection into rat gastrocnemius muscle. The investigators found that TTX produced a dose-dependent inhibition of mechanical hyperalgesia induced by the inflammogen carrageenan, which was still significant 24 hours after TTX administration. TTX was also shown to be effective in producing significant antinociceptive effect on muscle injury pain, by generating an increase in mechanical nociceptive threshold of exercise-induced mechanical hyperalgesia of the gastrocnemius muscle.[21]

NOVEL LOCAL ANESTHETIC DELIVERY SYSTEMS

Another approach in extending the effective therapeutic duration of LAs is via a novel delivery system. Recently, much attention has been focused on loading LAs into biomaterial-based carriers, such as nanoparticles or liposomes microparticles, to enhance the duration and/or safety of LAs. The most popular delivery system so far is liposomal spheres loaded with LAs, with each sphere surrounded by a lipid bilayer that allows for controlled release of drug over time.[22] A randomized, double-blinded study comparing liposomal bupivacaine to plain bupivacaine in subjects undergoing mammoplasty found lower opioid use in the liposomal bupivacaine group at 24 and 48 hours postoperation, with no increased adverse effect, although there was also no statistically significant difference in the mean cumulative pain score between the liposomal bupivacaine group and the plain bupivacaine group.[23] Another phase 2 randomized, double-blinded study of wound infiltration of liposomal bupivacaine compared with plain bupivacaine in subjects receiving total knee arthroplasty found statistically significant lower pain score in the liposomal bupivacaine group as measured by the numeric rating scale (NRS) at rest (NRS-R) at all time points up to 5 days after surgery. However, there was no difference in the NRS with activity (NRS-A), and there was no significant difference in adverse events between the 2 groups.[24] Finally, an analysis examining pooled efficacy data reflected in cumulative pain score from 10 randomized double-blinded phase II and phase III liposome bupivacaine clinical studies found that, when administered via local wound infiltration, liposomal bupivacaine produces lower cumulative pain scores up to 24 to 72 hours postsurgery compared with plain bupivacaine. However, there was no statistical difference in the requirement of rescue opioids between the liposomal bupivacaine group and plain bupivacaine. Overall, all 10 studies showed that liposome bupivacaine was well-tolerated and had an adverse event profile that was similar to plain bupivacaine.[25] A cost-benefit analysis on patients undergoing total knee arthroplasty found that significantly higher percentage of patients who received liposomal bupivacaine were able to ambulate on the day of surgery, walked further in the first 2 postoperative days, and were able to be discharged within 2 days after surgery.[26] Other retrospective studies have also shown that the average hospitalization cost of patients undergoing primarily total knee arthroplasty was lower in groups that had received periarticular infiltration of liposomal bupivacaine versus groups that had received femoral nerve block.[27,28] Finally, studies in patients undergoing laparoscopic hand-assisted nephrectomy or robotic-assisted hysterectomy have shown lower maximal postoperative pain score and decreased total opioid use with the use of liposomal bupivacaine in transverse abdominis plane (TAP) block, as compared to TAP block using plain bupivacaine.[29,30] Ultimately, while the efficacy of liposomal bupivacaine for the management of postoperative pain remains uncertain due to the small sample size and inconsistency of results in many of the available studies,[31,32] further research should allow us to elucidate any potential promise that liposomal bupivacaine may have when used in peripheral nerve blocks.

To further improve the safety profile and duration of action of STX, there also has been interest in encapsulating STX within liposomes, similar to the approaches previously outlined with LAs. For instance, injection of liposomal STX in Sprague-Dawley rats produced sciatic nerve blockade of between 13.5 hours to 48 hours, without signs of systemic toxicity; in addition, coincorporation of dexamethasone within liposomes produced blocks lasting up to 7.5 days without signs of toxicity.[33] Although transient mild to moderate focal inflammation were noted up to 4 days after local injection of liposomes, these reactions subsequently resolved by day 21, and no myotoxicity or neurotoxicity were seen in any formation that did not contain LAs. Another potential application of liposomal STX is in the treatment of neuropathic pain secondary to peripheral nerve injury. In studies using rats undergoing spared nerve injury, injection of liposomes containing both STX and dexamethasone delayed the onset of allodynia by 2 days, and treatment with 3 sequential injections produced a nerve block duration of 18 days and delayed the onset of allodynia by 1 month.[34] This is in contrast to application of bupivacaine and dexamethasone microspheres, which did not seem to have an effect on the development of allodynia or hyperalgesia in animals with spared nerve injury.[35] Similar to the first study, even multiple injections of STX and dexamethasone liposomes did not produce significant myotoxicity or neurotoxicity. Finally, the use of special liposome with gold nanomaterials has been studied as a method to enable in vivo repeated and on-demand anesthesia. Specifically, in an animal study, gold nanorods-conjugated liposomes containing TTX and dexmedetomidine were injected into the hindpaws of rats and near-infrared (NIR) light was used to heat the liposomes, which in turn increased membrane permeability and enabled triggered drug release. Through this novel method, the investigators were able to achieve repeatable triggered LA release by varying the amount and duration of NIR light radiation, without observing significant tissue inflammation or injury.[36] In another animal study, liposome incorporating a specially designed NIR-absorbing photosensitizer octabutoxyphthalocyaninato-palladium(II), $PdPC(OBu)_8$ and containing TTX were injected onto the sciatic nerve of rats. In this study, irradiation of injected site triggered controlled releases of TTX that returned to baseline after 2 hours and also produced a corresponding nerve block that was repeatable. Similar to the previous study, the level of inflammation and myotoxicity was low in and around the sciatic nerve injection site in both the treatment and control groups.[37]

Although liposomal LAs appear quite promising in clinical studies, their shelf-life is usually less than 1 to 2 months secondary to leakage of drug from the liposomes. Currently, proliposomal ropivacaine formulation that leads to liposomal formation only when in contact with aqueous subcutaneous tissue is in development. In an in vitro porcine wound healing study, exposure to saline and plasma effectively transformed the homogenous proliposomal oil into a liposomal emulsion, and proliposomal ropivacaine was able to provide sensory anesthesia for approximately 30 hours (vs 6 hours for plain ropivacaine), without additional adverse effects. In addition, the proliposomal ropivacaine formulation was found to be stable for over 24 months in normal room temperature conditions.[38] In another randomized in vivo study using subcutaneous injection of proliposomal ropivacaine into healthy volunteers, proliposomal ropivacaine provided prolonged anesthesia to both pinprick and heat for 29 hours and 36 hours, respectively (vs 16 hours and 12 hours, respectively, with plain ropivacaine), without increased incidence of side effects.[39]

As an alternative to existing methods of regional nerve blockade, studies have examined the use of intravenous injection of magnetic nanoparticles (MNPs) associated with LAs together with external magnet applied over targeted sites to produce a regional block. An injection of ropivacaine-associated MNPs with magnet application at the ankle of rats significantly increased withdrawal latencies of affected extremity to noxious stimuli, whereas it had no effect on the contralateral extremity. The maximum plasma concentration of ropivacaine was also found to be significantly lower in animals injected with ropivacaine-associated MNPs compared with animals that had received injection of plain ropivacaine.[40]

Finally, another field of active development is hydrogels, which are crosslinked networks of hydrophilic polymers with very high water content. These polymers can be effective in controlling the release of drugs such as LAs. In particular, recent development of thermoresponsive and pH-sensitive hydrogels, which gel on exposure to physiologic temperature or pH, thereby localizing drug release to the point of application, opens up the possibility of sustained and targeted release of LAs.[41] For example, a group of investigators developed a hyaluronic acid-based gel with thermosensitive properties as a delivery vehicle for bupivacaine, and demonstrated that subcutaneous injection of the hydrogel in rats was able to produce sustained release of bupivacaine for up to 10 days without producing increased evidence of inflammation or discomfort.[42] Similarly, another group of investigators developed a thermogelling biodegradable composite hydrogel-nanoparticle lidocaine delivery system that was shown in vivo to be able to produce effective anesthesia for 360 minutes compared with 110 minutes for plain lidocaine solution.[43] In another study, a thermosensitive bupivacaine-loaded hydrogel system was examined using a rat sciatic nerve blockade model, and was able to produce nerve block of up to 9 hours.[44] Finally, iontophoresis of hydrogels, which is a noninvasive technique based on the application of a low density electric current to facilitate the release of drugs, has been shown in vitro to increase the permeation rate of prilocaine by 12-fold. It can potentially serve as a needle-free strategy to speed the onset and prolong the duration of local anesthesia.[45]

NOVEL ADJUVANTS OF LOCAL ANESTHETICS

Another approach to extend the duration of LAs is via an adjuvant agent. The use of adjuvants in regional and neuraxial blocks is a well-established practice, such as the addition of opioids, clonidine, dexamethasone, and epinephrine. More recently, other adjuncts have emerged. Magnesium has received an increased attention as an adjunct. Although the mechanism of analgesia produced by magnesium has not been fully elucidated, it is thought to be in part mediated through N-methyl-d-aspartate (NMDA) antagonism, leading to the inhibition of sensitization after tissue injury. In a randomized study of subjects who underwent arthroscopic rotator cuff repair, injection of 10% magnesium with bupivacaine resulted in longer duration of analgesia and significantly lower pain score at 12 hours compared with bupivacaine plus saline but did not have any effect on cumulative fentanyl consumption.[46] Another randomized study examined the efficacy of adding 150 mg of magnesium to bupivacaine in thoracic paravertebral block in subjects undergoing elective open thoracic surgery. It found that the group that received both bupivacaine and magnesium experienced, on average, 64 minutes longer sensory block; had less pain at 24 and 36 hours after surgery; demonstrated smaller morphine requirement over 48 hours; and exhibited better postoperative pulmonary function test results (ie, peak expiratory flow rate, forced expiratory volume in one second, and forced vital capacity) compared with the group that had only received bupivacaine.[47] This result mirrors another prospective randomized study evaluating magnesium as an adjuvant in supraclavicular brachial plexus block. In subjects undergoing elective forearm and hand surgeries, the addition of 150 mg of magnesium in ropivacaine injection produced longer motor and sensory block, lower need for rescue opioid, and lower pain score at 24 hours postoperatively compared with subjects who had only received ropivacaine in their brachial plexus block.[48] Finally, when used in transversus abdominis plane (TAP) block, the addition of 150 mg of magnesium with bupivacaine in women undergoing total abdominal hysterectomy produced lower pain score, prolonged duration of analgesia (by an average of 571 minutes), and required less rescue analgesic for up to 12 hours.[49] Similar results were also observed in subjects receiving TAP block for laparoscopic cholecystectomy.[50] It is reassuring that in all of the previous studies, no magnesium-associated toxicity was observed in the experimental groups.[46–49] However, it is also important to note that the efficacy of magnesium in enhancing LA regional block has not been universally demonstrated. An earlier study in rats found that, paradoxically, the magnesium actually diminished the duration of sciatic nerve block by lidocaine, bupivacaine, or ropivacaine.[51] Also, the addition of 50 mg of magnesium with ropivacaine as an adjuvant in caudal anesthesia in children receiving lower abdominal or penoscrotal surgery did not show any significant difference in postoperative pain scale, duration of analgesia, or analgesia requirement. The investigators theorized that the lack of effect may be in part due to insufficient dose used in their study.[52] Therefore, although most of the randomized studies have shown that magnesium can help extend the clinical effect of LAs when used as an adjuvant in various regional blocks, further studies are needed to better define the exact dosage of magnesium that would yield the greatest efficacy while minimizing potential side effects, especially in pediatric populations.

Another adjuvant to LAs that has received increased attention is dexmedetomidine, which is a highly selective alpha-2 adrenergic agonist with sedative, sympatholytic, and analgesic properties.[53] When used in obturator block in subjects receiving transurethral resection of bladder tumors, a randomized study found that 1 μg/kg of dexmedetomidine decreased the dosage of lidocaine required to achieve an adequate surgical block. There was no significant increase in adverse effects, such as bradycardia, delayed recovery, or nerve toxicity, in the dexmedetomidine group.[54] Another randomized controlled study comparing 2 doses of dexmedetomidine in combination with bupivacaine for caudal block in children receiving infraumbilical surgeries found that both 1 μg/kg and 2 μg/kg of dexmedetomidine extended the analgesia duration of bupivacaine, whereas the group receiving the 2 μg/kg of dexmedetomidine exhibited longer duration of analgesia and less requirement for rescue analgesics within 24 hours of operation. Notably, although there were no significant side effects observed in either the control or the 1 μg/kg dexmedetomidine group, 4 subjects in the 2 μg/kg dexmedetomidine group developed bradycardia, and 1 subjects developed hypotension that was correctable with fluid bolus and atropine.[55]

SUMMARY

Although traditional amide-based and ester-based LAs effectively block pain, their relatively short duration of action limits their analgesic effectiveness, especially at controlling postoperative pain. Alternative strategies of prolonging the duration of LAs have been investigated (**Table 1**). These include novel delivery systems, novel adjuvants, or substitution with site-1 sodium channel blockers. These strategies have

Table 1
Summary of studies

	Characteristics
Site-1 selective sodium channel blockers	
NeoSTX	Devoid of cardiotoxicity, reversible skeletal and respiratory muscle weakness. Less hypotension compared with TTX. Produces significantly longer block duration, lower median pain score, and no difference in serious adverse events compared with bupivacaine. The addition of epinephrine improves duration while decreasing systemic toxicity.
TTX	Minimal myotoxicity and neurotoxicity. Marked synergism with conventional LAs. Effective in reducing mechanical hyperalgesia.
Novel LAs delivery systems	
Liposomal bupivacaine	Lower opioid use and lower pain score compared with plain bupivacaine in regional anesthesia. Also resulted in lower hospitalization cost compared with femoral nerve block.
Liposomal STX	Produces prolonged blocks of between 2–18 d and delayed the onset of neuropathic pain.
NIR sensitive liposomal TTX	Repeatable trigger TTX release and nerve block without increased inflammation and myotoxicity.
Proliposomal ropivacaine	Prolonged anesthesia for approximately 30 h in both porcine and human studies. Significantly longer shelf life of 2 y (compared with 1–2 mo for liposomal bupivacaine).
Magnetic ropivacaine-associated nanoparticles	Selective regional block of noxious stimuli while decreasing systemic plasma concentration of ropivacaine.
Hydrogels	Thermosensitive and pH-sensitive hydrogels transforms on exposure to physiologic conditions, thereby allowing for sustained targeted exposure of LAs.
Novel adjuvants of LAs	
Magnesium	Longer duration of anesthesia, lower pain scores and, in some studies, lower opioid requirements when used in combination with bupivacaine.
Dexmedetomidine	1 μg/kg dose effective in extending the analgesia duration of bupivacaine and lidocaine, and produces no significant increase in adverse effects.

shown significant potential in decreasing postoperative pain, rescue opioid requirement, hospital length-of-stay, and overall health care cost, while retaining similar safety profiles compared to LAs. Novel LA delivery systems, such as NIR, sensitive liposomes, thermos-sensitive and pH-sensitive hydrogels, and proliposomes, carry the most promise for targeted delivery of prolonged regional anesthesia, while decreasing systemic toxicity. Proliposomes also present the potential advantage of lower cost by enabling significantly longer shelf life at room temperature as compared with traditional liposomes. Further randomized-controlled clinical studies are warranted to define the most efficacious method of administration and dosage to help minimize the side effects while maximizing the duration and efficacy of these novel approaches.

REFERENCES

1. Dib-Hajj SD, Black JA, Waxman SG. Voltage-gated sodium channels: therapeutic targets for pain. Pain Med 2009;10(7):1260–9.
2. Stainman AL, Seeman P. Different sites of membrane action for tetrodotoxin and lipid-soluable anesthetics. Can J Physiol Pharmacol 1975;53:513–24.
3. Adams HJ, Blair MRJ, Takman BH. The local anesthetic activity of tetrodotoxin alone and in combination with vasoconstrictors and local anesthetics. Anesth Analg 1976;55:568–73.
4. Cestele S, Catterall WA. Molecular mechanisms of neurotoxin action on voltage-gated sodium channels.pdf. Biochimie 2000;82:883–92.
5. Goldberg YP, MacFarlane J, MacDonald ML, et al. Loss-of-function mutations in the Nav1.7 gene underlie congenital indifference to pain in multiple human populations. Clin Genet 2007;71(4):311–9.
6. Møiniche S, Mikkelsen S, Wetterslev J, et al. A qualitative systematic review of incisional local anaesthesia for postoperative pain relief after abdominal operations. Br J Anaesth 1998;81(3):377–83.
7. Kohane DS, Lu NT, Gökgöl-Kline AC, et al. The local anesthetic properties and toxicity of saxitonin homologues for rat sciatic nerve block in vivo. Reg Anesth Pain Med 2000;25(1):52–9.
8. Strichartz G, Rando T, Hall S, et al. On the mechanism by which saxitoxin binds to and blocks sodium channels. Ann N Y Acad Sci 1986;479:96–112.
9. Rodriguez-Navarro AJ, Lagos N, Lagos M, et al. Neosaxitoxin as a local anesthetic: preliminary observations from a first human trial. Anesthesiology 2007;106(2):339–45.
10. Andrinolo D, Michea LF, Lagos N. Toxic effects, pharmacokinetics and clearance of saxitoxin, a component of paralytic shellfish poison (PSP), in cats. Toxicon 1999;37:447–64.
11. Wylie MC, Johnson VM, Carpino E, et al. Respiratory, neuromuscular, and cardiovascular effects of neosaxitoxin in isoflurane-anesthetized sheep. Reg Anesth Pain Med 2012;37(2):152–8.
12. Baer M, Best PM, Reuter H. Voltage-dependent action of tetrodotoxin in mammalian cardiac muscle. Nature 1976;263:344–5.
13. Kao CY. Pharmacology of tetrodotoxin and saxitoxin. Fed Proc 1972;31:1117–23.
14. Rodriguez-Navarro AJ, Lagos M, Figueroa C, et al. Potentiation of local anesthetic activity of neosaxitoxin with bupivacaine or epinephrine: development of a long-acting pain blocker. Neurotox Res 2009;16(4):408–15.
15. Rodríguez-Navarro AJ, Berde CB, Wiedmaier G, et al. Comparison of neosaxitoxin versus bupivacaine via port infiltration for postoperative analgesia following laparoscopic cholecystectomy. Reg Anesth Pain Med 2011;36(2):103–9.

16. Lobo K, Donado C, Cornelissen L, et al. A Phase 1, dose-escalation, double-blind, block-randomized, controlled trial of safety and efficacy of neosaxitoxin alone and in combination with 0.2% bupivacaine, with and without epinephrine, for cutaneous anesthesia. Anesthesiology 2015;123(4):873–85.
17. Benoit PW, Yagiela A, Fort NF. Pharmacologic correlation between local anesthetic-induced myotoxicity and disturbances of intracellular calcium distribution. Toxicol Appl Pharmacol 1980;52:187–98.
18. Padera RF, Tse JY, Bellas E, et al. Tetrodotoxin for prolonged local anesthesia with minimal myotoxicity. Muscle Nerve 2006;34(6):747–53.
19. Sakura S, Bollen AW, Ciriales R, et al. Local anesthetic neurotoxicity does not result from blockade of voltage-gated sodium channels. Anesth Analg 1995;81:338–46.
20. Kohane DS, Yieh J, Lu NT, et al. A re-examination of tetrodotoxin for prolonged duration local anesthesia. Anesthesiology 1998;89:119–31.
21. Alvarez P, Levine JD. Antihyperalgesic effect of tetrodotoxin in rat models of persistent muscle pain. Neuroscience 2015;311:499–507.
22. Mantripragada S. A lipid based depot (DepoFoam technology) for sustained release drug delivery. Prog Lipid Res 2002;41(5):392–406.
23. Smoot JD, Bergese SD, Onel E, et al. The efficacy and safety of DepoFoam bupivacaine in patients undergoing bilateral, cosmetic, submuscular augmentation mammaplasty: a randomized, double-blind, active-control study. Aesthet Surg J 2012;32(1):69–76.
24. Bramlett K, Onel E, Viscusi ER, et al. A randomized, double-blind, dose-ranging study comparing wound infiltration of DepoFoam bupivacaine, an extended-release liposomal bupivacaine, to bupivacaine HCl for postsurgical analgesia in total knee arthroplasty. Knee 2012;19(5):530–6.
25. Bergese SD, Ramamoorthy S, Patou G, et al. Efficacy profile of liposome bupivacaine, a novel formulation of bupivacaine for postsurgical analgesia. J Pain Res 2012;5:107–16.
26. Kirkness CS, Asche CV, Ren J, et al. Cost-benefit evaluation of liposomal bupivacaine in the management of patients undergoing total knee arthroplasty. Am J Health Syst Pharm 2016;73(9):e247–254.
27. Kirkness CS, Asche CV, Ren J, et al. Assessment of liposome bupivacaine infiltration versus continuous femoral nerve block for postsurgical analgesia following total knee arthroplasty: a retrospective cohort study. Curr Med Res Opin 2016; 32(10):1727–33.
28. Cien AJ, Penny PC, Horn BJ, et al. Comparison between liposomal bupivacaine and femoral nerve block in patients undergoing primary total knee arthroplasty. J Surg Orthop Adv 2015;24(4):225–9.
29. Hutchins JL, Kesha R, Blanco F, et al. Ultrasound-guided subcostal transverse abdominis plane blocks with liposomal bupivacaine vs. non-liposomal bupivacaine for postoperative pain control after laparoscopic hand-assisted donor nephrectomy: a prospective randomised observer-blinded study. Anaesthesia 2016;71(8):930–7.
30. Hutchins J, Delaney D, Vogel RI, et al. Ultrasound guided subcostal transverse abdominis plane (TAP) infiltration with liposomal bupivacaine for patients undergoing robotic assisted hysterectomy: a prospective randomized controlled study. Gynecol Oncol 2015;138(3):609–13.
31. Hamilton TW, Athanassoglou V, Trivella M, et al. Liposomal bupivacaine peripheral nerve block for the management of postoperative pain. Cochrane Database Syst Rev 2016;Issue 8. Art. No.: CD011476. http://dx.doi.org/10.1002/14651858.CD011476.pub2.

32. Tong YC, Kaye AD, Urman RD. Liposomal bupivacaine and clinical outcomes. Best Pract Res Clin Anaesthesiol 2014;28(1):15–27.
33. Epstein-Barash H, Shichor I, Kwon AH, et al. Prolonged duration local anesthesia with minimal toxicity. Proc Natl Acad Sci U S A 2009;106(17):7125–30.
34. Shankarappa SA, Tsui JH, Kim KN, et al. Prolonged nerve blockade delays the onset of neuropathic pain. Proc Natl Acad Sci U S A 2012;109(43):17555–60.
35. Suter MR, Papaloïzos M, Berde CB, et al. Development of neuropathic pain in the rat spared nerve injury model is not prevented by a peripheral nerve block. Anesthesiology 2003;99(6):1402–8.
36. Zhan C, Wang W, McAlvin JB, et al. Phototriggered local anesthesia. Nano Lett 2016;16(1):177–81.
37. Rwei AY, Lee JJ, Zhan C, et al. Repeatable and adjustable on-demand sciatic nerve block with phototriggerable liposomes. Proc Natl Acad Sci U S A 2015; 112(51):15719–24.
38. Davidson EM, Haroutounian S, Kagan L, et al. A novel proliposomal ropivacaine oil: pharmacokinetic-pharmacodynamic studies after subcutaneous administration in pigs. Anesth Analg 2016;122(5):1663–72.
39. Ginosar Y, Haroutounian S, Kagan L, et al. Proliposomal ropivacaine oil: pharmacokinetic and pharmacodynamic data after subcutaneous administration in volunteers. Anesth Analg 2016;122(5):1673–80.
40. Mantha VR, Nair HK, Venkataramanan R, et al. Nanoanesthesia: a novel, intravenous approach to ankle block in the rat by magnet-directed concentration of ropivacaine-associated nanoparticles. Anesth Analg 2014;118(6):1355–62.
41. Bagshaw KR, Hanenbaum CL, Carbone EJ, et al. Pain management via local anesthetics and responsive hydrogels. Ther Deliv 2015;6(2):165–76.
42. Seol D, Magnetta MJ, Ramakrishnan PS, et al. Biocompatibility and preclinical feasibility tests of a temperature-sensitive hydrogel for the purpose of surgical wound pain control and cartilage repair. J Biomed Mater Res B Appl Biomater 2013;101(8):1508–15.
43. Yin QQ, Wu L, Gou ML, et al. Long-lasting infiltration anaesthesia by lidocaine-loaded biodegradable nanoparticles in hydrogel in rats. Acta Anaesthesiol Scand 2009;53(9):1207–13.
44. Hoare T, Young S, Lawlor MW, et al. Thermoresponsive nanogels for prolonged duration local anesthesia. Acta Biomater 2012;8(10):3596–605.
45. Cubayachi C, Couto RO, de Gaitani CM, et al. Needle-free buccal anesthesia using iontophoresis and amino amide salts combined in a mucoadhesive formulation. Colloids Surf B Biointerfaces 2015;136:1193–201.
46. Lee AR, Yi HW, Chung IS, et al. Magnesium added to bupivacaine prolongs the duration of analgesia after interscalene nerve block. Can J Anaesth 2012;59(1):21–7.
47. Ammar AS, Mahmoud KM. Does the addition of magnesium to bupivacaine improve postoperative analgesia of ultrasound-guided thoracic paravertebral block in patients undergoing thoracic surgery? J Anesth 2014;28(1):58–63.
48. Mukherjee K, Das A, Basunia SR, et al. Evaluation of Magnesium as an adjuvant in Ropivacaine-induced supraclavicular brachial plexus block: A prospective, double-blinded randomized controlled study. J Res Pharm Pract 2014;3(4): 123–9.
49. Rana S, Verma RK, Singh J, et al. Magnesium sulphate as an adjuvant to bupivacaine in ultrasound-guided transversus abdominis plane block in patients scheduled for total abdominal hysterectomy under subarachnoid block. Indian J Anaesth 2016;60(3):174–9.

50. Al-Refaey K, Usama EM, Al-Hefnawey E. Adding magnesium sulfate to bupivacaine in transversus abdominis plane block for laparoscopic cholecystectomy: A single blinded randomized controlled trial. Saudi J Anaesth 2016;10(2):187–91.
51. Hung YC, Chen CY, Lirk P, et al. Magnesium sulfate diminishes the effects of amide local anesthetics in rat sciatic-nerve block. Reg Anesth Pain Med 2007; 32(4):288–95.
52. Birbicer H, Doruk N, Cinel I, et al. Could adding magnesium as adjuvant to ropivacaine in caudal anaesthesia improve postoperative pain control? Pediatr Surg Int 2007;23(2):195–8.
53. Cormack JR, Orme RM, Costello TG. The role of alpha2-agonists in neurosurgery. J Clin Neurosci 2005;12(4):375–8.
54. Lu Y, Sun J, Zhuang X, et al. Perineural dexmedetomidine as an adjuvant reduces the median effective concentration of lidocaine for obturator nerve blocking: a double-blinded randomized controlled trial. PLoS One 2016;11(6):e0158226.
55. Meenakshi Karuppiah NP, Shetty SR, Patla KP. Comparison between two doses of dexmedetomidine added to bupivacaine for caudal analgesia in paediatric infraumbilical surgeries. Indian J Anaesth 2016;60(6):409–14.

Pharmacology of Octreotide

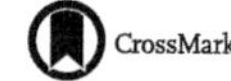

Clinical Implications for Anesthesiologists and Associated Risks

Reza M. Borna, MD[a,*], Jonathan S. Jahr, MD[a], Susanna Kmiecik, MD[a], Ken F. Mancuso, MD[b], Alan D. Kaye, MD, PhD, DABA, DABPM, DABIPP[b]

KEYWORDS

• Carcinoid syndrome • Carcinoid crisis • Octreotide • Sandostatin • Somatostatin

KEY POINTS

- Octreotide (Sandostatin, as octreotide acetate, Novartis Pharmaceuticals) is a longer acting synthetic octapeptide and analog of somatostatin, a naturally occurring hormone.
- Many patients presenting with a history of foregut, midgut neuroendocrine tumors or carcinoid syndrome can experience life-threatening carcinoid crises during anesthesia or surgery.
- Clinicians should understand the pharmacology of octreotide and appreciate the use of continuous infusions of high-dose octreotide, which can minimize the incidence of intraoperative carcinoid crises.

BACKGROUND

Octreotide (Sandostatin as octreotide acetate, Novartis Pharmaceuticals) is a longer acting synthetic octapeptide and analog of somatostatin, a naturally occurring hormone. The chemist Wilfried Bauer first synthesized octreotide in 1979.

CLINICAL PHARMACOLOGY

Octreotide acetate acts similar to somatostatin. It is an even more potent inhibitor of growth hormone, glucagon, and insulin. Somatostatin's inhibitory effects can be found throughout the human body, but particularly the endocrine and gastrointestinal

Disclosure Statement: None.
[a] Department of Anesthesiology and Perioperative Medicine, David Geffen School of Medicine at UCLA, Ronald Reagan UCLA Medical Center, 757 Westwood Plaza, Suite 3325, Los Angeles, CA 90095-7403, USA; [b] Department of Anesthesiology, LSUHSC, Room 656, 1542 Tulane Avenue, New Orleans, LA 70112, USA
* Corresponding author.
E-mail address: rborna@mednet.ucla.edu

Anesthesiology Clin 35 (2017) 327–339
http://dx.doi.org/10.1016/j.anclin.2017.01.021
1932-2275/17/Published by Elsevier Inc.

systems via neurotransmission and cell proliferation. In the hypothalamus, somatostatin inhibits the secretion of thyroid-stimulating hormone, growth hormone, adrenocorticotrophic hormone, and prolactin. It also inhibits the release of insulin, glucagon, gastrin, and other gastrointestinal peptides, thus reducing splanchnic blood flow, hepatic blood flow, and gastrointestinal motility, and increasing water and electrolyte absorption. Somatostatin is also an inhibitory neurotransmitter that inhibits cell proliferation.[1,2]

There are 5 subtypes of somatostatin receptors that have been identified. These 5 somatostatin receptors, referred to as sst1 through sst5, have been described as G-protein–coupled receptors. Of these receptors, most carcinoid tumors have a high concentration of type 2 receptors (sst2). Octreotide does not bind receptor types sst1 and sst4. However, receptor types sst2, sst3, and sst5 display a high, low, and moderate affinity, respectively, for the somatostatin analogs.[2,3]

PHARMACOKINETICS

Octreotide is absorbed poorly from the gut and thus it is administered parenterally. It is generally given as a subcutaneous bolus, although it can be given intravenously (IV) if a rapid effect is required.[1]

After subcutaneous injection, octreotide is absorbed rapidly and completely from the injection site. Peak concentrations of 5.2 ng/mL (100 μg dose) have been demonstrated 0.4 hours after dosing. Using a specific radioimmunoassay, IV and subcutaneous doses have been found to be bioequivalent. Peak concentrations and area under the curve values are dose proportional after IV single doses up to 200 μg and subcutaneous single doses up to 500 μg and after subcutaneous multiple doses up to 500 μg 3 times a day(1500 μg/d).[4]

The characteristics of octreotide include[4]:

- The distribution from plasma: rapid ($t\alpha 1/2 = 0.2$ h).
- Onset of action: 30 minutes.
- The volume of distribution (V_d): estimated to be 13.6 L, and the total body clearance ranged from 7 to 10 L/h.
- Time to peak plasma concentration: 30 minutes.
- Binding: mainly to lipoprotein and, to a lesser extent, to albumin.
- Metabolism: hepatic.
- The duration of action: variable, but extends up to 8 to 12 hours depending on the type of tumor.
- The elimination: has a half-life of 1.7 to 1.9 hours compared with 1 to 3 minutes with the natural hormone.
- Excretion: about 32% of the dose is excreted unchanged into the urine.
- Renal impairment: the elimination of octreotide from plasma is prolonged and total body clearance reduced.
  - In mild renal impairment (creatinine clearance 40–60 mL/min), the octreotide half-life is 2.4 hours and total body clearance is 8.8 L/h.
  - In moderate impairment (creatinine clearance 10–39 mL/min), the half-life is 3.0 hours and total body clearance 7.3 L/h.
  - In severely renally impaired patients not requiring dialysis (creatinine clearance <10 mL/min), the half-life is 3.1 hours and total body clearance is 7.6 L/h.
  - In patients with severe renal failure requiring dialysis, total body clearance is reduced to about one-half that found in healthy subjects (from approximately 10 to 4.5 L/h).

- In liver cirrhosis: prolonged elimination of drug, with octreotide half-life increasing to 3.7 hours and total body clearance decreasing to 5.9 L/h, whereas patients with fatty liver disease show half-life increases to 3.4 hours and total body clearance of 8.2 L/h.

FORMS

Octreotide Acetate

Injection is available as[4]:

- Sterile 1-mL ampules in 3 strengths
  - 50 μg
  - 100 μg
  - 500 μg
- Sterile 5-mL multidose vials in 2 strengths
  - 200 μg/mL
  - 1000 μg/mL

Octreotide Acetate Long-Acting Release

Octreotide acetate long-acting release is a depot formulation of octreotide, which is an injectable suspension. Octreotide acetate long-acting release has a relative bioavailability of 60% compared with subcutaneous octreotide. It is a 10- to 30-mg dose of octreotide given every 4 weeks and it comes in 3 strengths.[4]

- 10 mg per 6 mL
- 20 mg per 6 mL
- 30 mg per 6 mL

DOSAGE AND ADMINISTRATION

Octreotide may be administered subcutaneously or IV. Subcutaneous injection is the usual route of administration of octreotide acetate for control of symptoms. Pain with subcutaneous administration may be reduced by using the smallest volume that will deliver the desired dose. Multiple subcutaneous injections at the same site within short periods of time should be avoided. Sites should be rotated in a systematic manner.[4]

Octreotide is not compatible in total parenteral nutrition solutions because of the formation of a glycosyl octreotide conjugate, which may decrease the efficacy of the product.[4] Octreotide is stable in sterile isotonic saline solutions or sterile solutions of dextrose 5% in water for 24 hours. It may be diluted in volumes of 50 to 200 mL and infused IV over 15 to 30 minutes or administered by IV push over 3 minutes. In emergency situations (eg, carcinoid crisis), it may be given by rapid bolus.[4]

Dose varies according to the indication, although mostly it is recommended to titrate the dose to effect. The initial dosage is usually 50 μg administered 2 or 3 times daily. Upward dose titration is required frequently.[4]

DOSAGE FOR SPECIFIC CONDITIONS

Acromegaly

Dosage may be initiated at 50 μg 3 times a day. Beginning with this low dose may permit adaptation to adverse gastrointestinal effects for patients who require higher doses. The dose most commonly found to be effective is 100 μg 3 times a day, but some patients require up to 500 μg 3 times a day for maximum effectiveness.[4]

Carcinoid Tumors

The suggested daily dosage of octreotide during the first 2 weeks of therapy ranges from 100 to 600 μg/d in 2 to 4 divided doses (mean daily dosage is 300 μg).[4] Patients must be stabilized on subcutaneous octreotide for at least 2 weeks before switching to the intramuscular (IM) long-acting depot injection. Upon switch, a 20-mg IM dose is administered intragluteally every 4 weeks for 3 months, then the dose may be modified based on response. Patients should continue to receive their subcutaneous injections for the first 2 weeks at the same dose to maintain therapeutic levels (some patients may require 3–4 weeks of continued subcutaneous injections). Patients who experience periodic exacerbations of symptoms may require temporary subcutaneous injections in addition to depot injections (at their previous subcutaneous dosing regimen) until symptoms have resolved.[4]

Vasoactive Intestinal Peptide Tumors

Daily dosages of 200 to 300 μg in 2 to 4 divided doses are recommended during the initial 2 weeks of therapy (range 150–750 μg) to control symptoms of the disease.[4]

Carcinoid Crisis, Prevention

- Patients controlled with octreotide IM (depot) 20 to 30 mg: subcutaneously: 250 to 500 μg within 1 to 2 hours before the procedure.[5]
- Emergency surgery in somatostatin analog–naive patients with functional NETs: IV bolus 500 to 1000 μg 1 to 2 hours before the procedure or subcutaneously 500 μg 1 to 2 hours before the procedure.[5]
- Intraoperative use for carcinoid crisis with hypotension: IV 500 to 1000 μg bolus, repeat at 5-minute intervals until symptoms are controlled or IV 500 to 1000 μg bolus followed by 50 to 200 μg/h continuous infusion during the procedure.[5]
- Postoperative dose (if supplemental doses required during procedure): IV 50 to 200 μg/h continuous infusion for 24 hours, followed by resumption of the preoperative treatment schedule.[5]

Esophageal Varices Bleeding

As an IV bolus, give 25 to 100 μg (usual bolus dose is 50 μg) followed by a continuous IV infusion of 25 to 50 μg/h for 2 to 5 days. The bolus may be repeated in the first hour if the hemorrhage is not controlled.[6]

Malignant Bowel Obstruction

Give 200 to 900 μg/d subcutaneously in 2 to 3 divided doses[7] or 300 μg/d by continuous subcutaneously infusion.[8]

ROLE OF OCTREOTIDE IN MEDICINE

Because of somatostatin's broad effects throughout the body, octreotide has multiple therapeutic purposes. It is largely used in hormone-secreting tumors, such as carcinoid (inhibiting serotonin and thus improving flushing and diarrhea), vasoactive intestinal peptide tumors (inhibiting vasoactive intestinal peptide and decreasing diarrhea), and glucagonomas (inhibiting glucagon and improving rash and diarrhea).[1]

Acromegaly

Octreotide reduces blood levels of growth hormone and insulinlike growth factor-I (somatomedin C) in acromegaly patients who have had inadequate response to or cannot be treated with surgical resection, pituitary irradiation, or bromocriptine mesylate at maximally tolerated doses. Octreotide reduces growth hormone to within normal ranges in 50% of patients and reduces insulinlike growth factor-I to within normal ranges in 50% to 60% of patients. Improvement in clinical signs and symptoms or reduction in tumor size or rate of growth were not shown in clinical trials performed with octreotide.[4]

Carcinoid Tumors

Octreotide is indicated for the symptomatic treatment of patients with metastatic carcinoid tumors where it suppresses or inhibits the severe diarrhea and flushing episodes associated with the disease. Octreotide studies were not designed to show an effect on the size, rate of growth, or development of metastases.[4]

Vasoactive Intestinal Peptide Tumors

Octreotide is indicated for the treatment of the profuse watery diarrhea associated with vasoactive intestinal peptide-secreting tumors.[4]

Pain Control

Octreotide is reported to have an analgesic effect in patients with cancer, for example, in bone pain from metastatic carcinoid, in hypertrophic pulmonary osteoarthropathy or pain arising from GI cancer. However, a small randomized, controlled trial found octreotide to be no better than placebo.[9] Octreotide also is reported to be of value in chronic nonmalignant pancreatic pain caused by hypertension in the scarred pancreatic ducts. Benefit could be secondary to its antisecretory action.[1]

Esophageal Varices Bleeding

Octreotide causes splanchnic vasoconstriction at pharmacologic doses. Although it has been considered that this effect is due to an inhibition of the release of vasodilatory peptides (mainly glucagon), recent studies suggest that octreotide has a local vasoconstrictive effect.[6] Octreotide has been shown to prolong survival in patients with GI tract solid tumors owing to its direct anticancer effects.[1]

Malignant Bowel Obstruction

Octreotide can be used in inoperable bowel obstruction because it can provide rapid relief of nausea and vomiting.[1,7,8]

Refractory and Chylous Ascites

Octreotide is useful in patients with refractory ascites[1,10] and chylous ascites[11] of liver cirrhosis. Octreotide can suppress diuretic-induced activation of the renin–aldosterone–angiotensin system, causing improved renal function and sodium as well as water excretion.[1]

Off-Label Uses

- Carcinoid crisis (prevention)
- Diarrhea (refractory or persistent) associated with chemotherapy
- Diarrhea associated with graft-versus-host disease
- Gastroenteropancreatic NETs (metastatic)
- Hepatorenal syndrome
- Sulfonylurea-induced hypoglycemia
- Thymoma/thymic malignancies (advanced)
- AIDS-associated diarrhea (including cryptosporidiosis)
- Congenital hyperinsulinism
- Cushing's syndrome (ectopic)

- Hypothalamic obesity
- Postgastrectomy dumping syndrome
- Small bowel fistulas
- Zollinger-Ellison syndrome

NEW STUDIES AND NEW ROLES FOR OCTREOTIDE

Transfusion Requirements During Orthotopic Liver Transplantation

A recent investigation has evaluated the effects of continuous octreotide infusion on intraoperative transfusion requirements during orthotopic liver transplantation. The authors have hypothesized that intraoperative transfusion requirements would be reduced in those patients treated with octreotide.[12] Although this small study did not show a statistical difference in the number of units transfused, there was an absolute difference. A prospective, randomized trial would be useful in elucidating the true effect of octreotide on red blood cell transfusion requirements during orthotopic liver transplantation.[12]

Postoperative Chylothorax

Chylothorax is an extremely rare and serious complication of cardiac surgery. In a recent study by Owais and colleagues, the investigators report a case of a 76-year-old woman who developed chylothorax after coronary artery bypass grafting. The chylothorax was successfully treated in 7 days by octreotide administration and medium-chain triglycerides enriched diet. Based on this study, octreotide is an effective, valid, and safe drug for the treatment of postoperative chylothorax and may highly reduce the need for reoperation.[13]

CONTRAINDICATIONS

There is no contraindication for the usage of octreotide, unless the patient has sensitivity to the drug or any of its components.[4]

ANESTHETIC CONSIDERATIONS

The role of octreotide largely has been studied in the setting of carcinoid tumors and carcinoid syndrome. These tumors are responsible for the secretion of a variety of hormones, including serotonin, bradykinins, prostaglandins, vasoactive peptide, and histamine, which are responsible for the presentation of carcinoid syndrome.[14]

Carcinoid tumors are rare, slow-growing neoplasms of neuroendocrine tissues from enterochromaffin or Kulchitsky cells, which have the potential to metastasize. The mediators released from these tumors—serotonin, histamine, and the kinins—bypass the hepatic metabolism and lead to development of the carcinoid syndrome. This is a life-threatening complication, which can lead to profound hemodynamic instability, especially in a perioperative period, when the patient is exposed to various types of noxious stimuli.[2,15]

Carcinoid syndrome is characterized by flushing, bronchoconstriction, diarrhea, and at times with significant hemodynamic instability often termed carcinoid crisis. It is hypothesized that a carcinoid crisis event can happen when there is a sudden catecholamine-mediated surge of hormones, which when bypassing portal circulation and thus metabolism, can cause major hemodynamic shifts and life-threatening symptoms. This theory regarding a catecholamine-mediated response has caused some practitioners to avoid medications, which may promote this unwanted effect.[2,14]

Treatment depends on the type, location, and stage of the tumor. Complete surgical excision of the tumor is the most effective treatment, which may be a partial bowel resection and mesenteric lymphadenectomy. Some metastatic lesions can also be removed surgically. Octreotide can also be used to treat the symptoms produced by any residual tumor left after surgery. Hepatic metastasis can be dealt with hepatic artery occlusion by ligation, embolization and transarterial chemoembolization.[2,15]

The goal of perioperative management is to avoid carcinoid crisis by preventing the release of bioactive mediators. Life-threatening complication with hemodynamic instability can occur in a perioperative period when the patient is exposed to various types of noxious stimuli, which can lead to significant morbidity and mortality.

Special perioperative and preanesthetic planning is required for the patient presenting with a NET, largely related to concern for carcinoid crisis. A stress response owing to anesthetic or surgical stimuli may cause release of vasoactive substances, resulting in significant hemodynamic instability unresponsive to conventional therapies.[14]

Preoperative Evaluation and Optimization

Preoperative assessment includes the following.

- Detailed history and physical examination for determining the presence and severity of any symptoms of carcinoid syndrome.
- A complete cardiac evaluation, including electrocardiogram and echocardiography.

Preoperative optimization of patient's general condition and underlying pathology for surgery play a major role. Malnutrition, dehydration, anemia, and electrolyte imbalance related to diarrhea and to intestinal obstruction are common findings. Symptoms and signs of on-going uncontrolled hormonal activity may be present. Unpredictable, uncontrolled release of hormones precipitated by any stimulation such as variation of hemodynamics parameters, anesthetic agents or surgical stimuli can occur, which may result in hypertensive or hypotensive crisis and hemodynamic collapse, which may be unresponsive to conventional drug therapy. Thus, it is very important to minimize tumor activity before commencing surgery.

Somatostatin analogs have become the mainstay of medical therapy, especially in patients whose disease is beyond resection with curative intent.[16] Octreotide has almost replaced all other drugs used for carcinoid patients. No standard octreotide administration regimen is reliable, and various recommendations have been proposed. Ideally, it should be started at the dose of 100 μg 3 times daily and 100 μg just before induction to suppress sudden release of mediators. It should be administered in infusion at 50 μg/h for at least 12 hours before surgery.[15]

Preoperative therapy is aimed at optimization of the patient for surgery and providing relief of symptoms. This goal may be achieved by antagonizing the mediators of carcinoid syndrome or by blocking their release. Since its introduction, octreotide has become the mainstay of therapy.[17]

Several drugs block the production, release, or action of mediators from these tumors. Of the mediators released from carcinoid tumors, the easiest to antagonize is histamine. The effects of histamine are blocked by antihistamines such as chlorpheniramine, and histamine-2 blockers such as ranitidine. Aprotinin, a kallikrein inhibitor, has been used to treat flushing associated with bradykinin production.[2]

Anesthetic Techniques

Although virtually all patients with carcinoid tumor are operated under a general anesthetic technique to avoid sympathectomy by neuraxial anesthesia, both spinal and epidural anesthesia have been used successfully.[18] Preoperative use of octreotide, judicious fluid therapy, and low-dose local anesthetics with low-dose opioids have made neuraxial block possible. Moreover, an epidural catheter can be used for postoperative analgesia. total intravenous anesthesia with propofol and remifentanil has been demonstrated to be successful, particularly for abdominal surgery. Its major advantages are hemodynamic stability, significantly shorter times of emergence, and exceptional acceptance by patients[19]; results have revealed a clinically significant reduction of postoperative nausea and vomiting compared with isoflurane–nitrous oxide anesthesia[15]

For conventional general anesthesia, similarly the primary aim is to provide stability and controlled environment in these operations, which may take as little as 5 to 6 hours or as long as 10 to 15 hours. The keys for achieving this state are adequate depth, good analgesia, and avoidance of drugs that stimulate the release of vasoactive mediators such as morphine and atracurium. All emergency drugs should be kept ready for any untoward event. IV boluses of 20 to 25 μg of octreotide can be used to treat the release of mediators intraoperatively. Vasopressin is an alternative treatment.[15]

Postoperative Care

These patients are very prone to delayed emergence from anesthesia related to high levels of serotonin. All standard monitoring used intraoperatively should be continued in the postoperative period as well. Particular care should be exercised while managing morbidly obese patients. The mediators may continue to exert their effects after removal of the tumor and some occult tumor may continue to produce mediators. Hence, these patients need to be monitored in intensive care units or, minimally, high-dependency units. Octreotide therapy should be continued, which can be slowly tapered off over 1 week, according each patient's response. Good analgesia plays a major role in preventing any excess sympathetic activity and stress. This can be achieved by epidural analgesia or IV fentanyl infusion. Dexmedetomidine is a newer agent in anesthesia practice that can be used effectively for sedation and augmentation of postoperative analgesia.[20] Serotonin-induced hyperglycemia should be monitored and controlled with insulin infusion (**Table 1**).

OCTREOTIDE USE DURING ANESTHESIA

Unfortunately, the literature is sparse in terms of exact octreotide implications and its dosage in anesthesia management; the available data are limited by few studies and case reports. The burden is mostly left to the physicians' judgment based on the drug's pharmacodynamics and interactions on each patient's individual basis.

- Octreotide dosages of 250 to 500 μg subcutaneously can be given to the patient controlled with octreotide IM (depot) within 1 to 2 hours before the procedure.[5]
- In emergency surgeries, IV bolus of 500 to 1000 μg or 500 μg subcutaneously 1 to 2 hours, before a procedure should be considered.[5]
- For carcinoid crisis with hypotension, a 500- to 1000-μg IV bolus, repeated at 5-minute intervals, until symptoms are controlled or 500 to 1000 μg IV bolus, followed by 50 to 200 μg/h continuous infusion during the procedure is recommended.[5]
- There are new studies that have shown that octreotide infusions do not prevent intraoperative crises.[21] Based on these results, the decision to use the infusion for the prevention of crisis has become somewhat more controversial, although most practices continue to use octreotide.
- If supplemental doses are required during a procedure, octreotide should be continued in the postoperative period at 50 to 200 μg/h continuous infusion for 24 hours, followed by resumption of the preoperative treatment schedule.[5]

Table 1
Anesthesia for carcinoid syndrome

Concern	Comment
Preoperative	
Diarrhea	Dehydration, electrolyte abnormalities.
Tricuspid regurgitation or pulmonary stenosis	Right heart failure.
Hyperglycemia	
Hypoalbuminemia	
Premedication	
Octreotide	0.1–1.0 mg IV + 100–500 μg/h infusion.
Antihistamines	H_1 and H_2 blockers (diphenhydramine [Benadryl], famotidine [Pepcid AC]).
Antibiotics	
Hydrocortisone	Might be considered for patients with very high 5-hydroxy indole acetic acid levels, who are continuously flushed.
Intraoperative	
Octreotide	Infusion continues at the rate ordered and started in preoperatively.
No histamine releasers	Avoid medications like morphine, meperidine (Demerol), and atracurium.
Intubation and maintenance	• Avoid stressful or light intubation. • Fentanyl, propofol, etomidate, and volatile anesthetics are safe. • Use rocuronium or vecuronium for relaxation.
Hypertension	For hypertension not owing to light anesthesia, consider beta blockers like labetalol.
Hypotension	• Use crystalloid or colloid. • Administer octreotide, especially if flushing or bronchospasm presents. • No ephedrine or epinephrine (can precipitate serotonergic crisis).
PONV	Ondansetron (Zofran) can be given for antiemetic; plus, it is an 5-HT antagonist.
Postoperative	
Octreotide	Continue infusion, which can be slowly tapered off over 1 wk.
Monitoring	• All standard monitoring should be continued. • Patients should be monitored in intensive care units or minimally, high dependency units.
Pain control	• Epidural analgesia. • Intravenous fentanyl infusion. • PCA. • Dexmedetomidine can be used for sedation and augmentation of postoperative analgesia.
Serotonin-induced hyperglycemia	Should be monitored and controlled with insulin infusion.

Abbreviations: PCA, patient-controlled analgesia; PONV, postoperative nausea and vomiting.

CARCINOID CRISIS: IS IT PREVENTABLE?

A carcinoid crisis is a serious and potentially life-threatening exacerbation of the carcinoid syndrome, characterized by profound flushing, bronchospasm, tachycardia, and widely fluctuating blood pressure. Patients with either midgut (small bowel, appendix, right colon) or foregut (respiratory tract, thymus, stomach, duodenum, pancreatic) NETs are at risk for experiencing a carcinoid crisis during anesthesia, surgery, or radiologic interventions regardless of whether or not they have been diagnosed as having the carcinoid syndrome.[14]

Because of its potential to present in the operative period, the use of octreotide to prevent or treat during surgery has been studied.

- Massimino and colleagues[22] found that prevention of carcinoid crisis with a 500-μg bolus of octreotide acetate preoperatively was unsuccessful. In their study, 19% of patients experiences prolonged (>10 minutes) hypotension with an additional 5% exhibiting hemodynamic instability consistent with carcinoid crisis. It is postulated that octreotide's limited plasma half-life of 90 to 120 minutes possibly limits its usefulness in prophylaxis against carcinoid crisis because blood concentration would decrease to below 50% after 2 hours and consequently to 25% within 4 hours.[14]
- Condron and colleagues[21] also found that carcinoid crisis prophylaxis in patients with known carcinoid tumors with an octreotide bolus 500 μg followed by infusion at 500 μg/h did not prevent a crisis event (30% crisis rate for infusion group as compared with 24% in bolus alone).
- Another recent study done by Kaye and colleagues, at Louisiana State University has shown that a 500 μg/h infusion of octreotide acetate preoperatively, intraoperatively, and postoperatively minimizes the incidence of carcinoid crisis. In their study, the incidence of crisis was just 3.4%.[14]

Despite competing and inconsistent data, related to its overall low cost and excellent safety profile, many institutions continue the use of octreotide as bolus and infusion in the perioperative setting to prevent a carcinoid crisis during the debulking and resection of NETs.[14]

DRUG INTERACTIONS

Octreotide has been associated with alterations in nutrient absorption; therefore, it may have an effect on absorption of orally administered drugs. In this regard, concomitant administration of octreotide with cyclosporine may decrease blood levels of cyclosporine and result in transplant rejection.[4]

Additionally, patients receiving insulin, oral hypoglycemic agents, beta blockers, calcium channel blockers, or agents to control fluid and electrolyte balance may require dose adjustments of these therapeutic agents.[4]

CAUTIONS

- Octreotide should be used cautiously in the setting of insulinoma and blood glucose control in diabetics because it can lower glucose levels drastically and reduce insulin requirements by up to 50%. Plasma glucose concentrations should be monitored carefully during octreotide use.[4]
- Octreotide can increase the bioavailability of bromocriptine by up to 40%, which should be considered because both drugs are used in the treatment of acromegaly.[4]
- Octreotide may cause bradycardia, arrhythmias, or conduction defects and should be used with caution in at-risk patients.[4]

SIDE EFFECTS

1. Gallbladder abnormalities, especially stones and biliary sludge.[1,4]
2. Cardiac
   - Bradycardia develops in 25% of acromegalics.
   - Conduction abnormalities (10%).
   - Arrhythmias (9%).
3. Gastrointestinal (34%–61%)
   - Diarrhea.
   - Nausea.
   - Abdominal discomfort.
4. Dermatologic: pruritus (≤18%).
5. Hypoglycemia (3%) and hyperglycemia (16%).
6. Hypothyroidism: In acromegalics, biochemical hypothyroidism alone occurred in 12% and goiter occurred in 6% during octreotide acetate. In patients without acromegaly, hypothyroidism has only been reported in several isolated patients and goiter has not been reported.
7. Pain on injection (7.7%).
8. Headache and dizziness (6%).
9. Other side effects, which happen in fewer than 4% of patients on octreotide, include fatigue, weakness, pruritus, joint pain, backache, urinary tract infection, cold symptoms, flu symptoms, injection site hematoma, bruise, edema, flushing, blurred vision, pollakiuria, fat malabsorption, hair loss, visual disturbance, and depression.

OCTREOTIDE AND PREGNANCY

Octreotide is considered a category B medication, which means that animal reproduction studies have failed to demonstrate a risk to the fetus and there are no adequate and well-controlled studies in pregnant women. Reproduction studies have been performed in rats and rabbits at doses up to 16 times the highest recommended human dose based on body surface area and revealed no evidence of harm to the fetus owing to octreotide. However, because animal reproduction studies are not always predictive of human response, this drug should be used during pregnancy only if clearly needed.[4]

OCTREOTIDE AND BREAST FEEDING

It is not known whether octreotide is excreted into human milk. Because many drugs are excreted in human milk, caution should be exercised when octreotide is administered to a nursing woman.[4]

OCTREOTIDE AND PEDIATRIC USE

No formal controlled clinical trials have been performed to evaluate the safety and effectiveness of octreotide in pediatric patients under age 6 years. In postmarketing reports, serious adverse events, including hypoxia, necrotizing enterocolitis, and death, have been reported with octreotide use in children, most notably in children under 2 years of age. The relationship of these events to octreotide has not been established because the majority of these pediatric patients had serious underlying comorbid conditions.[4]

OCTREOTIDE AND GERIATRIC USE

Clinical studies of octreotide have not included sufficient numbers of subjects aged 65 and older to determine whether geriatric patients respond differently from younger subjects. Other reported clinical experiences have not identified differences in responses between elderly and younger patients. In general, dose selection for an elderly patient should be cautious, usually starting at the low end of the dosing range, reflecting the greater frequency of decreased hepatic, renal, and cardiac function, and of concomitant disease or other drug therapy.[4,8]

Many patients presenting with a history of foregut, midgut NETs, or carcinoid syndrome can experience life-threatening carcinoid crises during anesthesia or surgery. Clinicians should understand the pharmacology of octreotide and appreciate the use of continuous infusions of high dose octreotide, which can minimize the incidence of intraoperative carcinoid crises. At our Louisiana State University facility, where patients have surgery daily, we administer a prophylactic 500-μg bolus of octreotide IV and begin a continuous infusion of 500 μg/h for all NET patients during surgery, regardless of the location of their primary tumor or functional status. Advantages of octreotide include low cost of an infusion and excellent safety profile.

SUMMARY

The use of infusions of high-dose octreotide during extensive debulking procedures for midgut and foregut NETs require anesthesiologists to appreciate the pathophysiology involved in the disease process, the pharmacology of this agent, drug–drug interactions, and potential side effects.

REFERENCES

1. Wilcock A, Twycross R. Therapeutic reviews: octreotide. J Pain Symptom Manage 2010;40(1):142–8.
2. Mancuso K, Kaye AD, Boudreaux JP, et al. Carcinoid syndrome and perioperative anesthetic considerations. J Clin Anesth 2011;23:329–41.
3. Dierdorf S. Carcinoid tumor and carcinoid syndrome. Curr Opin Anaesthesiol 2003;16:343–7.
4. Sandostatin, Octreotide acetate injection; Prescribing Information. Novartis Pharmaceuticals Corporation; 2012.
5. Oberg K, Kvols L, Caplin M, et al. Consensus report on the use of somatostatin analogs for the management of neuroendocrine tumors of the gastroenteropancreatic system. Ann Oncol 2004;15(6):966–73.
6. Garcia-Tsao G, Bosch J. Management of varices and variceal hemorrhage in cirrhosis. N Engl J Med 2010;362:823–32.
7. Mercadante S, Porzio G. Octreotide for malignant bowel obstruction: twenty years after. Crit Rev Oncol Hematol 2012;83(3):388–92.
8. Ripamonti C, Mercadante S, Groff L, et al. Role of Octreotide, scopolamine butylbromide, and hydration in symptom control of patients with inoperable bowel obstruction and nasogastric tubes: a prospective randomized trial. J Pain Symptom Manage 2000;19(1):23–34.
9. De Conno F, Saita L, Ripamonti C, et al. Subcutaneous octreotide in the treatment of pain in advanced cancer patients. J Pain Symptom Manage 1994;9:34–8.
10. Kalambokis G, Fotopoulos A, Economou M, et al. Octreotide in the treatment of refractory ascites of cirrhosis. Scand J Gastroenterol 2006;41(1):118–21.
11. Zhou DX, Zhou HB, Wang Q, et al. The effectiveness of the treatment of octreotide on chylous ascites after liver cirrhosis. Dig Dis Sci 2009;54(8):1783–8.
12. Byram SW, Gupta RA, Ander M, et al. Effects of continuous octreotide infusion on intraoperative transfusion requirements during orthotopic liver transplantation. Transplant Proc 2015;47(9):2712–4.

13. Owais TA, Back D, Girdauskas E, et al. Postoperative chylothorax: is octreotide a valid therapy? J Case Rep Stud 2015;3(3):307.
14. Woltering EA, Wright AE, Stevens MA, et al. Development of effective prophylaxis against intraoperative carcinoid crisis. J Clin Anesth 2016;32:189–93.
15. Bajwa SJ, Panda A, Kaur G. Carcinoid tumors: challenges and considerations during anesthetic management. J Scientific Soc 2015;V42(3):132–7. Available at: http://www.jscisociety.com/article.asp?issn=0974-5009;year=2015;volume=42;issue=3;spage=132;epage=137;aulast=Bajwa.
16. Bendelow J, Apps E, Jones LE, et al. Carcinoid syndrome. Eur J Surg Oncol 2008;34:289–96.
17. Vaughan DJ, Brunner MD. Anesthesia for patients with carcinoid syndrome. Int Anesthesiol Clin 1997;35:129–42.
18. Orbach-Zinger S, Lombroso R, Eidelman LA. Uneventful spinal anesthesia for a patient with carcinoid syndrome managed with long-acting octreotide. Can J Anaesth 2002;49:678–81.
19. Farling PA, Durairaju AK. Remifentanil and anaesthesia for carcinoid syndrome. Br J Anaesth 2004;92:893–5.
20. Bajwa S, Kulshrestha A. Dexmedetomidine: an adjuvant making large inroads into clinical practice. Ann Med Health Sci Res 2013;3:475–83.
21. Condron ME, Pommier SJ, Pommier RF. Continuous infusion of octreotide combined with perioperative octreotide bolus does not prevent intraoperative carcinoid crisis. Surgery 2015;159(1):358–67.
22. Massimino K, Harrskog O, Pommier S, et al. Octreotide LAR and bolus octreotide are insufficient for preventing intraoperative complications in carcinoid patients. J Surg Oncol 2013;107(8):842–6.

An Analysis of New Approaches and Drug Formulations for Treatment of Chronic Low Back Pain

CrossMark

Karishma Patel Bhangare, MD[a],
Alan D. Kaye, MD, PhD, DABA, DABPM, DABIPP[b],
Nebojsa Nick Knezevic, MD, PhD[c], Kenneth D. Candido, MD[c],
Richard D. Urman, MD, MBA[a,*]

KEYWORDS

- Chronic low back pain • Chemonucleolysis • Platelet-rich plasma injections
- Artemin • Tanezumab • Stem cells • Matrix metalloproteinases • Ethanol
- Collagenase

KEY POINTS

- The prevalence of chronic low back pain (CLBP) is increasing. Treatment for the disorder is effective in less than 50% of patients after 1 year.
- The safety and efficacy of new treatments for CLBP over the previous 3-year period are evaluated and described in detail in this review.
- This investigation identified new treatments for CLBP, including chemonucleolysis (using collagenase, chondroitinase ABC, matrix metalloproteinases, and ethanol gel), platelet-rich plasma injections, artemin, tanezumab, and stem cells.
- Further research and innovation are needed to implement these methods into practice and assess clinical significance. Current evidence suggests promising new agents for the treatment of CLBP.

INTRODUCTION

With our aging, overweight, and overworked population, chronic low back pain (CLBP) will continue to be one of the most common chief complaints that results in a patient

Disclosure Statement: The authors have nothing to disclose.
[a] Department of Anesthesiology, Perioperative and Pain Medicine, Brigham and Women's Hospital, Harvard Medical School, 75 Francis Street, Boston, MA 02115, USA; [b] Department of Anesthesiology and Pain Medicine, Louisiana State University School of Medicine, LSU Health Science Center, 1542 Tulane Avenue, Room 659, New Orleans, LA 70112, USA; [c] Department of Anesthesiology and Pain Medicine, Advocate Illinois Masonic Medical Center, 836 West Wellington Avenue, Suite 4815, Chicago, IL 60657, USA
* Corresponding author.
E-mail address: urmanr@gmail.com

Anesthesiology Clin 35 (2017) 341–350
http://dx.doi.org/10.1016/j.anclin.2017.01.023
anesthesiology.theclinics.com
1932-2275/17/

visiting a pain physician. In this regard, its prevalence has increased from 3.9% in 1992 to 10.2% in 2006.[1] With more diagnostic tests and therapeutic interventions available, the total cost related to CLBP in the United States is now greater than $100 billion per year.[2] Workers' compensation expenditure for musculoskeletal disease, mainly low back pain, is greater than $20 billion per year on its own.[2] The cost is also increasing for employers; an estimated 101.8 million days of work are lost each year secondary to low back pain.[3] This results in decreased productivity and lost wages. By the time an employee has been out of work for 6 months, the likelihood of him or her ever returning to work is 50%. Nevertheless, the prognosis for CLBP is promising. Costa and colleagues[4] found that 47% of patients with CLBP had recovered by 12 months. Therefore, it is prudent that these patients receive appropriate and efficacious treatment early. Pain physicians play a large part in propelling patients to go back to work, live an active lifestyle, carry out activities of daily living, and improve psychological well-being. This review article aims to discuss new approaches and treatment options on the horizon for the treatment of CLBP.

Anatomy and Pathophysiology

There are numerous causes of CLBP, with the most recognized being degeneration and herniation of intervertebral discs (IVDs). Each IVD is composed of a nucleus pulposus (NP) surrounded by an annulus fibrosus (AF). The NP is a gelatinous inner core composed of type II collagen, proteoglycans, and noncollagenous proteins.[5] Glycosaminoglycans and hyaluronic acid chains are linked to the proteoglycans. The NP acts as a "shock absorber." It transmits radial pressure onto the vertebral endplates to reduce internal friction.[6] The AF has fibroblasts that synthesize types I and II collagen into circumferential rings. This orientation gives it the ability to provide tensile strength and resist anterior and posterior sliding of vertebral bodies.[6] Between the vertebral body and the IVD is a thin layer of hyaline cartilage. Also known as the endplate, its function is to distribute intradiscal pressures onto adjacent vertebrae to prevent the NP from bulging into underlying trabecular bone.[7]

In a normal IVD, the synthesis and degradation of tissues are balanced. However, when nutrient supply decreases and/or cellular demand increases, degradation predominates and the disc loses its biomechanical function.[8,9] IVDs are predominantly avascular.[10] Consequently, nutrient supply becomes an issue. The AF receives nutrients from nearby capillaries. Inner disc cells rely on nutrient diffusion from capillaries off vertebral bodies that terminate near the endplates.[11] During times of high disc degeneration, growth factors and cytokines are expressed.[12] This increases glucose consumption and lactic acid production. Nutrient demand increases, which a cell may not be able to keep up with, resulting in more disc degeneration.[13] As the balance is further skewed, proteoglycans and glycosaminoglycans are lost and type II collagen denatures.[14] The discs dehydrate and are more likely to herniate.[15] Furthermore, a decrease in disc height increases loading on nearby joints, resulting in osteoarthritic changes and thickening of the ligamentum flavum.[16,17]

CURRENT TREATMENTS

In 2007, the American College of Physicians and the American Pain Society formulated joint clinical practice guidelines for the diagnosis and treatment of low back pain. Conservative nonpharmacologic treatment includes physical therapy, acupuncture, chiropractic manipulations, yoga, Tai Chi, cognitive behavioral therapy, and meditation.[18] Conservative pharmacologic treatment includes acetaminophen, nonsteroidal antiinflammatory drugs, muscle relaxants, opioids, tramadol, and tricyclic antidepressants. If conservative treatment fails, invasive treatment is considered. This includes epidural steroid injections, spinal cord stimulators, and spine surgery.

Chemonucleolysis

Chymopapain has been identified to be effective in vivo for enzymatic intradiscal therapy. It is a catalyst for the cleavage of glycosaminoglycans from proteoglycan aggregates in the disc. These reactions decrease the water-binding capacity of the polysaccharide side chains.[19] As a result of decreased disc pressure, disc protrusion decreases and there is less tension on nerve roots.[20] Adverse reactions of chymopapain include anaphylaxis, discitis, subarachnoid hemorrhage, paraplegia, and acute transverse myelitis. Consequently, chymopapain was withdrawn from the market in the early 2000s.

Collagenase

The potential risks have generated interest in other enzymes with less allergic potential, such as collagenase. Collagenase splits type II collagen fibers. Wittenberg and colleagues[21] performed a 5-year clinical follow-up assessment of a prospective, randomized study to compare the efficacy of chymopapain and collagenase for intradiscal injection. The investigators randomized 100 patients to treatment with either 4000 IU of chymopapain or 400 ABC units of collagenase. Inclusion criteria included sciatic leg pain stronger than back pain and a 6-week minimum of unsuccessful conservative treatment. Exclusion criteria included neurologic deficits, pregnancy, allergy to injection substance, and surgery at the same segment. The disc injection was performed with fluoroscopic control under general anesthesia. After discharge, the patients were seen after 2, 6, and 12 weeks and then for a 1-year, 3-year, and 5-year follow-up visits. Of the patients in the chymopapain group, 12% showed allergic reactions. Of these, 1 patient had an anaphylactic reaction. At each time interval, patients rated their results as excellent, good, fair, or poor. Those lost to follow-up or those who underwent surgery were rated poor. In the chymopapain group, 72% rated the results as excellent or good at 5 years and 52% in the collagenase group. Pain scales decreased from 8.5 to 0.7 in the chymopapain group and 8.6 to 0.9 in the collagenase group. Patients in the chymopapain group returned to work in 8 weeks and those in the collagenase group returned to work in 11 weeks. The authors concluded that both substances are not significantly different. However, chymopapain is known to be relatively safe, whereas collagenase needs further studies.

Chondroitinase ABC

Chondroitinase ABC (C-ABC) is another enzyme that has been reported to be as efficacious as chymopapain.[22] However, there was no study that assessed intradiscal pressure changes from C-ABC in vivo. Sasaki and colleagues[23] took 11 sheep and injected different doses of C-ABC into several IVDs. Phosphate-buffered saline was injected in the control group. Intradiscal pressure was measured using a pressure transducer 1 week before injection and then at 1 and 4 weeks after injection. Disc height index was measured by roentgenograms at the same time intervals. The authors found that low dose C-ABC (1 and 5 U) induced a small decrease in intradiscal pressure at 1 week and a greater reduction at 4 weeks. High dose C-ABC (50 U) induced a statistically significant effect after 1 week and a greater decrease at 4 weeks. There was no change in intradiscal pressure over time in the control group. The disc height index decreased more in the low-dose C-ABC group than the high-dose group. There was no correlation found between the decrease in intradiscal pressure and disc height index (r = 0.339). Accordingly, using disc height as a surrogate for intradiscal pressure to evaluate chemonucleolysis may be inaccurate.

Matrix Metalloproteinases

Matrix metalloproteinases (MMPs) are a family of proteolytic enzymes that participate in the degradation of matrix components such as glycoproteins, proteoglycans, and collagen. MMP-3 degrades the protein core of proteoglycans and small noncollagenous proteins. Their activity is inhibited by tissue inhibitors of metalloproteinases (TIMPs). It has been hypothesized that the dysbalance of MMPs and TIMPs leads to disc degeneration. Bachmeier and colleagues[24] took 37 lumbar specimens obtained during operative procedures such as lumbar discectomies and interbody fusions. The control group was composed of samples taken from healthy polytrauma patients where discs were removed for surgical stabilization. A quantitative molecular analysis of the messenger RNA expression for MMPs and TIMPs was performed using reverse transcriptase polymerase chain reaction. The researchers found that MMP-3 messenger RNA levels were upregulated consistently in samples with histologic evidence of disc degeneration. Interestingly, TIMP-1 was also upregulated. The authors concluded that MMP-3 plays a key role in the degenerative cascade leading to symptomatic disc herniation. Gaining control of this enzyme may be a new treatment for IVD disease.

In 2005, Haro and colleagues[25] conducted an extensive study to examine the role of MMPs in the treatment of herniated discs. Five disc samples were taken from patients undergoing primary lumbar herniotomy. The tissues were cultured without recombinant human (rh) MMP-3, with rh MMP-3, with rh MMP-7, and with chymopapain. They were later stained with safranin O, which is an indicator for proteoglycan content. In addition, rh MMP-3, rh MMP-7, and chymopapain were injected into healthy disc tissue of 5 Japanese white rabbits. One week later, disc samples were taken, fixed, and stained with safranin O. In the final group, 10 beagles suffering from herniated discs were given either rh MMP-7, chymopapain, or saline. Safranin O staining was performed and MRI and myelography were done to investigate morphologic changes. The authors found that culturing human surgical tissue with rh MMP-3, rh MMP-7, and chymopapain resulted in strong degradation of proteoglycans. Similar results were seen in the healthy rabbit IVDs. The level of degradation was greatest with rh MMP-7 and chymopapain. Administration of rh MMP-7 and chymopapain into canine herniated discs resulted in a decrease in protruded disc mass as seen by MRI and myelography. Histologically, rh MMP-7 destroyed the NP, but an intact nucleus area and AF remained. In contrast, chymopapain showed degradation through the NP and AF. This potentially could allow the disc chondrocytes to regenerate the NP in rh MMP-7–treated cells, but not in chymopapain treated cells. The authors concluded that rh MMP-7 shows the greatest promise for the treatment of herniated discs.

With the results discussed, Haro and colleagues[26] further studied the effects of rh MMP-7 using human herniated discs in vitro and dogs in vivo. Surgical samples of herniated discs obtained during patients undergoing primary lumbar herniotomy were taken and incubated with or without rh MMP-7. The wet weight and concentration of keratan sulfate was measured before and after treatment. Keratan sulfate is a degradation product of IVDs. The wet weight of herniated discs decreased in a concentration-dependent manner and the keratan sulfate level increased. When patient age, grade of herniation, and interval between onset of symptoms and surgery were controlled for, there was no correlation between the decrease in wet weight and any of these associated conditions. Hence, rh MMP-7 may be used for a wide range of patients with herniated discs. To study its effect in vivo, 20 male beagles were anesthetized and injected with rh MMP-7 into lumbar IVDs. After 1 week, injected discs were harvested and stained to examine proteoglycan content and keratan sulfate concentration. Proteoglycan content decreased in a dose-dependent manner and the keratan sulfate concentration increased. [125I]-labeled rhMMP-7 injected into lumbar IVDs in canines showed radioactivity in the NP and AF, but not in muscle and surrounding tissue. No rh MMP-7 changes were noted in clinical signs, body weight, food consumption, or necropsy findings to suggest systemic effects.

Ethanol

Chemonucleolysis by ethanol is another potential treatment for CLBP. Bellini and colleagues[27] enrolled 90 patients with lumbar or cervical disc herniations. They were treated with intradiscal injections of radiopaque gelified ethanol. Radiopaque gelified ethanol causes dehydration of the NP resulting in disc herniation retraction. Inclusion criteria included disc herniation contained, without complete annulus tear, and not contained, with posterior longitudinal ligament integrity and no free fragments assessed with MRI or computed tomography. Exclusion criteria included previous surgery at the symptomatic level, high degree of disc degeneration, spinal stenosis, and asymptomatic disc bulging. Pain was evaluated by the visual analog scale (VAS) and Oswestry Disability Index immediately after treatment and then in 3 months. Eighty-five percent of patients with lumbar disc herniation and 83% of patients with cervical disc herniation obtained significant symptom improvement. The VAS score decreased by 4 points and Oswestry Disability Index decreased by 40%. Leakage of radiopaque gelified ethanol to surrounding tissue occurred in 19 patients without any clinical side effects. Touraine and colleagues[28] found similar results with percutaneous chemonucleolysis using ethanol gel in patients who failed conservative treatment. Pain intensity decreased by 44% after 1 month and 62% after 3 months (P = .007). The VAS score decreased from 7 at baseline to 3.8 at 1 month and 2.6 at 3 months (P<.0001). The authors of both studies concluded that ethanol is safe and effective in reducing the symptoms of disc herniation.

Platelet-Rich Plasma Injections

Platelet-rich plasma (PRP) is obtained by concentrating platelets and other blood components from an autologous sample of blood. The platelets, growth factors, and cytokines in the concentrate increase collagen content, accelerate endothelial regeneration, and promote angiogenesis.[29] Levi and colleagues[30] took 22 patients with discogenic pain defined as positive discography, clinical features suggestive of discogenic pain, and features of discogenic pain on MRI and injected intradiscal PRP. The VAS was assessed before treatment and 1, 2, and 6 months after treatment. At 6 months, 9 out of 19 patients had a 50% improvement in symptoms and there was a 50% decrease in the VAS. A prospective, double-blinded, randomized, controlled study was done in 2016 to determine whether PRP injections improved pain and function in symptomatic degenerative IVDs.[31] Fifty-eight patients who met the trial criteria were included in the study. Thirty-six patients were in the treatment group and 22 were in the control group. The patients were followed for 1 year using several different metrics including the Functional Rating Index, Numeric Rating Scale, 36-Item Short Form Health Survey, and patient satisfaction (North American Spine Society Outcome Questionnaire). Over the first 8 weeks, there were statistically significant improvements in the Numeric Rating Scale (P = .20), Functional Rating Index (P = .03), and North American Spine Society Outcome Questionnaire (P = .10). These improvements were maintained in the 1-year follow-up period. Neither study reported any complications after the intradiscal injection of PRP.

Artemin

Artemin is a member of the glial cell line-derived neurotrophic factor family of ligands.[32] It binds to the GFRα3 receptor on the RET receptor tyrosine kinase.[33] This receptor is expressed after axonal damage.[34] Artemin promotes survival of sensory, sympathetic, and central neurons. Several animal studies have found artemin to prevent histochemical changes in the dorsal root ganglion, maintain C-fiber function, and restore sensory neuron function after nerve injury.[35] Subjects with unilateral sciatica for at least 6 weeks and a pain rating of 40 mm or greater on the 100-mm VAS were included in a study by Rolan and colleagues.[36] The participants were divided into 11 groups: placebo and different doses of intravenous and subcutaneous artemin. Assessments were done at baseline and then after treatment at 15 minutes, 1 hour, 6 hours, 24 hours, 72 hours, and 28 days. Pain was graded using the VAS and Likert scale. There were no dose-dependent trends in the VAS or Likert scale. Adverse events included heat intolerance, pruritus, headache, and rash. The incidence was higher at doses 100 μg/kg or greater. There were no dose-dependent trends related to vital signs, laboratory parameters, intraepidermal nerve fiber density, or quantitative sensory testing. Artemin antibodies were detected in 2 subjects in the treatment group, but both had negative results in a subsequent assay for neutralizing antibodies. The authors believe that no trend was seen regarding efficacy because it was not the study's primary outcome, the patients were on concomitant analgesic therapy, and the sample size was small. Because the medication is safe and tolerable, the researchers support the continued clinical development of this agent for treatment of neuropathic pain.

Tanezumab

Neurotrophin nerve growth factor (NGF) is a key mediator of the generation and potentiation of pain signals in tissue injury.[37] Increased NGF levels are associated with increased pain perception in several chronic pain conditions.[38] Tanezumab is a high-affinity monoclonal antibody against NGF. It prevents NGF from binding to tropomyosin-related kinase A and p75.[39] It has been shown to reduce chronic pain from osteoarthritis, CLBP, and interstitial cystitis.[40–42] To confirm and extend those findings, Kivitz and colleagues[43] studied tanezumab's efficacy and safety. The investigators enrolled 1347 patients in the study. Inclusion criteria included CLBP 3 or more months requiring short-acting analgesic medications, average low back pain intensity (LBPI) score of 4 or greater, and Patient Global Assessment of the low back as fair, poor, or very poor. Exclusion criteria included back surgery in the past 6 months; significant cardiac, neurologic, or other pain; psychological conditions; and long-acting opioids within 3 months. Subjects were randomized to placebo, naproxen (500 mg 2 times per day by mouth), tanezumab (intravenously every 8 weeks) 5 mg, 10 mg, and 20 mg. Pain was assessed at weeks 2, 4, 8, 12, 16, and 24. Efficacy was measured by the LBPI score, Roland-Morris Disability Questionnaire score, and Patient Global Assessment. At 16 weeks, the 20-mg tanezumab group had a mean LBPI change from baseline of −2.18 versus −0.93 in the placebo group ($P<.001$) and −0.5 in the naproxen group ($P = .006$). Tanezumab 10 mg resulted in a similar mean change from baseline. However, tanezumab 5 mg did not reach statistical significance compared with placebo or naproxen. A similar pattern was seen when the Roland-Morris Disability Questionnaire was performed. Using the Patient Global Assessment, tanezumab 20 mg, 10 mg, and 5 mg had a statistically significant difference between treatment and placebo. The maximum reduction of LBPI score was seen at 4 weeks and maintained over the course of the study. Frequent adverse events in the treatment group included paresthesia, arthralgia, pain in extremity, headache, hyperesthesia, dysesthesia, and osteonecrosis.

Stem Cell Therapy

Regenerative cellular therapy has been a large focus of research over the past decade. It has the potential to increase synthesis of proteoglycans and type II collagen for IVD rebuilding. There are multiple cell sources that differentiate into chondrocyte-like cells including mesenchymal stem cells (MSCs), embryonic stem cells, induced pluripotent stem cells, human umbilical cord MSCs, and NP cells.[44] MSCs have been differentiated into chondrocyte-like cells in vitro and in vivo.[45,46]

Transplantation of MSCs in animal degenerated IVD models showed survival of chondrocyte-like cells.[47] These cells were capable of aggrecan production, leading to an increase in IVD height.[47] In humans, injection of MSCs into the NP of an affected segment showed an increase in NP water content.[48] Subjects reported rapid improvement in pain and functional status.[48] Anatomically, studies have shown IVD height and disc height index increase in MSC transplant groups.[49] Histologically, transplantation decreases degeneration grading scale values.[50] Furthermore, MRI shows water content increases in the treated NP.[51] Molecularly, MSC-treated NPs have an increase in type II collagen messenger RNA.[52] MSCs have antiinflammatory effects and can reverse fibrosis by secretion of cytokines and MMPs.[53]

Orozco and colleagues[48] injected autologous expanded bone marrow MSCs in the NP of 10 patients with CLBP from lumbar disc degeneration. The patients were followed for 1 year and analyzed by the VAS, Oswestry Disability Index, and 36-Item Short Form Health Survey. MRI measurements of disc height and fluid content were also done. There was a rapid improvement in pain and disability at 3 months followed by modest additional improvements at 12 months. Water content increased, but disc height did not recover. No major adverse effects were recorded.

Injectate extravasation includes major risks such as discitis, tumorigenesis, osteophytes, and spinal stenosis. Subhan and colleagues[54] studied carriers to limit stem cell extravasation. Rabbits with iatrogenic disc damage were given MSCs in HyStem (hyaluronan-based hydrogel), HyStem alone, and no intervention. After 8 weeks, histologic analysis and MRI was done. HyStem hydrogel with MSCs had a high T2-weighted signal intensity suggesting increased disc water content, high height index, low degenerative index, and more type II collagen and aggrecan staining. Although many studies are preliminary, further work is being conducted as regenerative cellular therapy can have a profound impact on future treatment of damaged IVDs.

SUMMARY

The IVD has a limited vascular supply, which makes it a poor environment for healing from herniation or degeneration. Chemonucleolysis via collagenase, C-ABC, MMP, and ethanol gel have shown improvements in CLBP symptomatology. Further studies are being conducted with MMP-7 and ethanol gel. Growth factors such as PRP, artemin, and tanezumab have shown various levels of CLBP improvement. More research is needed to assess their safety and clinical effectiveness. Stem cell treatment has shown significant improvement in pain scores and disability. Further clinical trials are underway to evaluate the safety and efficacy.

REFERENCES

1. Freburger JK, Holmes GM, Agans RP, et al. The rising prevalence of chronic low back pain. Arch Intern Med 2009;169(3):251–8.

2. Katz JN. Lumbar disc disorders and low-back pain: socioeconomic factors and consequences. J Bone Joint Surg Am 2006;88(Suppl 2):21–4.
3. Guo HR, Tanaka S, Halperin WE, et al. Back pain prevalence in US industry and estimates of lost workdays. Am J Public Health 1999;89(7):1029–35.
4. Costa Lda C, Maher CG, McAuley JH, et al. Prognosis for patients with chronic low back pain: inception cohort study. BMJ 2009;339:b3829.
5. Hooten WM, Cohen SP. Evaluation and treatment of low back pain: a clinically focused review for primary care specialists. Mayo Clin Proc 2015;90(12): 1699–718.
6. Vora AJ, Doerr KD, Wolfer LR. Functional anatomy and pathophysiology of axial low back pain: disc, posterior elements, sacroiliac joint, and associated pain generators. Phys Med Rehabil Clin N Am 2010;21(4):679–709.
7. Brinckmann P, Frobin W, Hierholzer E, et al. Deformation of the vertebral endplate under axial loading of the spine. Spine (Phila Pa 1976) 1983;8(8):851–6.
8. Huang YC, Urban JP, Luk KD. Intervertebral disc regeneration: do nutrients lead the way? Nat Rev Rheumatol 2014;10(9):561–6.
9. Sivan SS, Hayes AJ, Wachtel E, et al. Biochemical composition and turnover of the extracellular matrix of the normal and degenerate intervertebral disc. Eur Spine J 2014;23(Suppl 3):S344–53.
10. Grunhagen T, Shirazi-Adl A, Fairbank JC, et al. Intervertebral disk nutrition: a review of factors influencing concentrations of nutrients and metabolites. Orthop Clin North Am 2011;42(4):465–77, vii.
11. Roberts S, Menage J, Urban JP. Biochemical and structural properties of the cartilage end-plate and its relation to the intervertebral disc. Spine (Phila Pa 1976) 1989;14(2):166–74.
12. Risbud MV, Shapiro IM. Role of cytokines in intervertebral disc degeneration: pain and disc content. Nat Rev Rheumatol 2014;10(1):44–56.
13. Shirazi-Adl A, Taheri M, Urban JP. Analysis of cell viability in intervertebral disc: effect of endplate permeability on cell population. J Biomech 2010;43(7):1330–6.
14. Antoniou J, Steffen T, Nelson F, et al. The human lumbar intervertebral disc: evidence for changes in the biosynthesis and denaturation of the extracellular matrix with growth, maturation, ageing, and degeneration. J Clin Invest 1996;98(4): 996–1003.
15. Urban JP, Roberts S. Degeneration of the intervertebral disc. Arthritis Res Ther 2003;5(3):120–30.
16. Adams MA, Dolan P, Hutton WC, et al. Diurnal changes in spinal mechanics and their clinical significance. J Bone Joint Surg Br 1990;72(2):266–70.
17. Postacchini F, Gumina S, Cinotti G, et al. Ligamenta flava in lumbar disc herniation and spinal stenosis. Light and electron microscopic morphology. Spine (Phila Pa 1976) 1994;19(8):917–22.
18. Chou R, Qaseem A, Snow V, et al, Clinical efficacy assessment subcommittee of the American College of Physicians, American College of Physicians; American Pain Society Low Back Pain Guidelines Panel. Diagnosis and treatment of low back pain: a joint clinical practice guideline from the American College of Physicians and the American Pain Society. Ann Intern Med 2007;147(7):478–91.
19. Smith L. Enzyme dissolution of the nucleus pulposus in humans. JAMA 1964;187: 137–40.
20. Suguro T, Oegema TR Jr, Bradford DS. The effects of chymopapain on prolapsed human intervertebral disc. A clinical and correlative histochemical study. Clin Orthop Relat Res 1986;(213):223–31.

21. Wittenberg RH, Oppel S, Rubenthaler FA, et al. Five-year results from chemonucleolysis with chymopapain or collagenase: a prospective randomized study. Spine (Phila Pa 1976) 2001;26(17):1835–41.
22. Ando T, Kato F, Mimatsu K, et al. Effects of chondroitinase ABC on degenerative intervertebral discs. Clin Orthop Relat Res 1995;(318):214–21.
23. Sasaki M, Takahashi T, Miyahara K, et al. Effects of chondroitinase ABC on intradiscal pressure in sheep: an in vivo study. Spine (Phila Pa 1976) 2001;26(5): 463–8.
24. Bachmeier BE, Nerlich A, Mittermaier N, et al. Matrix metalloproteinase expression levels suggest distinct enzyme roles during lumbar disc herniation and degeneration. Eur Spine J 2009;18(11):1573–86.
25. Haro H, Komori H, Kato T, et al. Experimental studies on the effects of recombinant human matrix metalloproteinases on herniated disc tissues–how to facilitate the natural resorption process of herniated discs. J Orthop Res 2005;23(2): 412–9.
26. Haro H, Nishiga M, Ishii D, et al. Experimental chemonucleolysis with recombinant human matrix metalloproteinase 7 in human herniated discs and dogs. Spine J 2014;14(7):1280–90.
27. Bellini M, Romano DG, Leonini S, et al. Percutaneous injection of radiopaque gelified ethanol for the treatment of lumbar and cervical intervertebral disk herniations: experience and clinical outcome in 80 patients. AJNR Am J Neuroradiol 2015;36(3):600–5.
28. Touraine S, Damiano J, Tran O, et al. Cohort study of lumbar percutaneous chemonucleolysis using ethanol gel in sciatica refractory to conservative treatment. Eur Radiol 2015;25(11):3390–7.
29. Podd D. Platelet-rich plasma therapy: origins and applications investigated. JAAPA 2012;25(6):44–9.
30. Levi D, Horn S, Tyszko S, et al. Intradiscal platelet-rich plasma injection for chronic discogenic low back pain: preliminary results from a prospective trial. Pain Med 2016;17(6):1010–22.
31. Tuakli-Wosornu YA, Terry A, Boachie-Adjei K, et al. Lumbar intradiskal platelet-rich plasma (PRP) injections: a prospective, double-blind, randomized controlled study. PM R 2016;8(1):1–10.
32. Airaksinen MS, Saarma M. The GDNF family: signalling, biological functions and therapeutic value. Nat Rev Neurosci 2002;3:383–94.
33. Baloh RH, Tansey MG, Lampe PA, et al. Artemin, a novel member of the GDNF ligand family, supports peripheral and central neurons and signals through the GFRalpha3-RET receptor complex. Neuron 1998;21:1291–302.
34. Bennett DL, Boucher TJ, Armanini MP, et al. The glial cell line-derived neurotrophic factor family receptor components are differentially regulated within sensory neurons after nerve injury. J Neurosci 2000;20:427–37.
35. Bennett DL, Boucher TJ, Michael GJ, et al. Artemin has potent neurotrophic actions on injured C-fibres. J Peripher Nerv Syst 2006;11:330–45.
36. Rolan PE, O'Neill G, Versage E, et al. First-in-human, double-blind, placebo-controlled, randomized, dose-escalation study of BG00010, a Glial cell line-derived neurotrophic factor family member, in subjects with unilateral sciatica. PLoS One 2015;10(5):e0125034.
37. Frade JM, Barde YA. Nerve growth factor: two receptors, multiple functions. Bioessays 1998;20:137–45.
38. Watson JJ, Allen SJ, Dawbarn D. Targeting nerve growth factor in pain: what is the therapeutic potential? BioDrugs 2008;22:349–59.

39. Abdiche YN, Malashock DS, Pons J. Probing the binding mechanism and affinity of tanezumab, a recombinant humanized anti-NGF monoclonal antibody, using a repertoire of biosensors. Protein Sci 2008;17:1326–35.
40. Brown M, Murphy F, Radin D, et al. Tanezumab reduces osteoarthritic knee pain: results of a randomized, double-blind, placebo-controlled phase 3 trial. J Pain 2012;13:790–8.
41. Katz N, Borenstein DG, Birbara C, et al. Efficacy and safety of tanezumab in the treatment of chronic low back pain. Pain 2011;152:2248–58.
42. Evans RJ, Moldwin RM, Cossons N, et al. Proof of concept trial of tanezumab for the treatment of symptoms associated with interstitial cystitis. J Urol 2011;185: 1716–21.
43. Kivitz AJ, Gimbel JS, Bramson C, et al. Efficacy and safety of tanezumab versus naproxen in the treatment of chronic low back pain. Pain 2013;154(7):1009–21.
44. Gou S, Oxentenko SC, Eldrige JS, et al. Stem cell therapy for intervertebral disk regeneration. Am J Phys Med Rehabil 2014;93(11 Suppl 3):S122–31.
45. Kim DH, Kim SH, Heo SJ, et al. Enhanced differentiation of mesenchymal stem cells into NP-like cells via 3D co-culturing with mechanical stimulation. J Biosci Bioeng 2009;108:63–7.
46. Wei A, Chung SA, Tao H, et al. Differentiation of rodent bone marrow mesenchymal stem cells into intervertebral disc-like cells following coculture with rat disc tissue. Tissue Eng Part A 2009;15:2581–95.
47. Ho G, Leung VY, Cheung KM, et al. Effect of severity of intervertebral disc injury on mesenchymal stem cell-based regeneration. Connect Tissue Res 2008;49: 15–21.
48. Orozco L, Soler R, Morera C, et al. Intervertebral disc repair by autologous mesenchymal bone marrow cells: a pilot study. Transplantation 2011;92(7): 822–8.
49. Yang F, Leung VYL, Luk KDK, et al. Mesenchymal stem cells arrest intervertebral disc degeneration through chondrocytic differentiation and stimulation of endogenous cells. Mol Ther 2009;17:1959–66.
50. Sakai D, Mochida J, Iwashina T, et al. Regenerative effects of transplanting mesenchymal stem cells embedded in atelocollagen to the degenerated intervertebral disc. Biomaterials 2006;27:335–45.
51. Bendtsen M, Bunger CE, Zou X, et al. Autologous stem cell therapy maintains vertebral blood flow and contrast diffusion through the endplate in experimental intervertebral disc degeneration. Spine (Phila Pa 1976) 2011;36:E373–9.
52. Sakai D, Mochida J, Iwashina T, et al. Differentiation of mesenchymal stem cells transplanted to a rabbit degenerative disc model: potential and limitations for stem cell therapy in disc regeneration. Spine 2005;30:2379–87.
53. Leung V, Aladin D, Lv F, et al. Mesenchymal stem cells mediate disk regeneration by suppression of fibrosis in nucleus pulposus. Global Spine J 2012;2:1.
54. Subhan RA, Puvanan K, Murali MR, et al. Fluoroscopy assisted minimally invasive transplantation of allogenic mesenchymal stromal cells embedded in HyStem reduces the progression of nucleus pulposus degeneration in the damaged intervertebral disc: a preliminary study in rabbits. ScientificWorldJournal 2014;2014: 818502.

Index

Note: Page numbers of article titles are in **boldface** type.

Anesthesiology Clin 35 (2017) 351–363
http://dx.doi.org/10.1016/S1932-2275(17)30038-1
1932-2275/17

C

F

G

H

O

P

R

S

T

U

V

W

X

Moving?

Make sure your subscription moves with you!

To notify us of your new address, find your **Clinics Account Number** (located on your mailing label above your name), and contact customer service at:

Email: journalscustomerservice-usa@elsevier.com

800-654-2452 (subscribers in the U.S. & Canada)
314-447-8871 (subscribers outside of the U.S. & Canada)

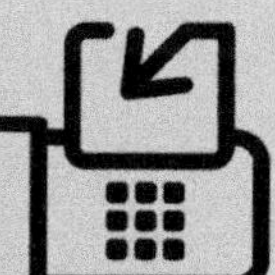

Fax number: 314-447-8029

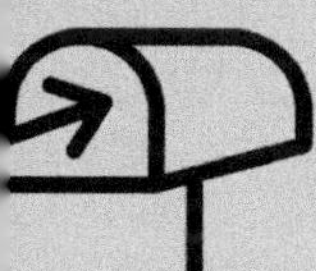

Elsevier Health Sciences Division
Subscription Customer Service
3251 Riverport Lane
Maryland Heights, MO 63043

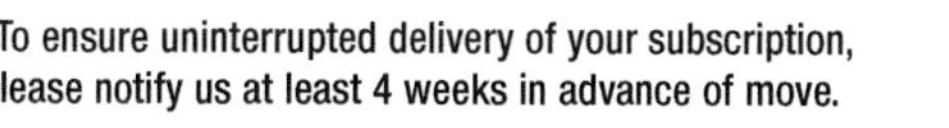

*To ensure uninterrupted delivery of your subscription, please notify us at least 4 weeks in advance of move.

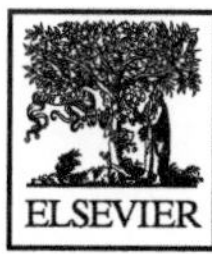

Printed and bound by CPI Group (UK) Ltd, Croydon, CR0 4YY

08/05/2025

01864699-0010